Care Boss

Leadership Strategies & Resources for Family Caregivers

JENNIFER A. O'BRIEN, MSOD

Award-winning author of *The Hospice Doctor's Widow*

— WISE INK MEDIA —
MINNEAPOLIS, MN

Care Boss © copyright 2024 by Jennifer A. O'Brien
All rights reserved. No part of this book may be reproduced in any form whatsoever, by photography or xerography or by any other means, by broadcast or transmission, by translation into any kind of language, nor by recording electronically or otherwise, without permission in writing from the author, except by a reviewer, who may quote brief passages in critical articles or reviews.

ISBN 13: 978-1-63489-741-9
Library of Congress Catalog Number has been applied for.
Printed in the United States of America
First Printing: 2024
28 27 26 25 24   5 4 3 2 1

Cover design by Jennifer A. O'Brien
Interior design by Vivian Steckline
Author photo by Lori Sparkman
Edited by Carolyn Williams-Noren
Proofread by Chelsey Burden and Elizabeth Farry
Production editing by Victoria Petelin

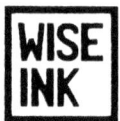

Wise Ink
PO Box 580195
Minneapolis, MN 55458-0195
www.WiseInk.com

Wise Ink is a creative publishing agency for game-changers. Wise Ink authors uplift, inspire, and inform, and their titles support building a better and more equitable world. For more information, visit WiseInk.com.

To order, visit JenniferAOBrien.com. Reseller discounts available.

Contact Jennifer A. O'Brien at JenniferAOBrien.com for speaking engagements, freelance writing projects, and interviews.

Praise for Care Boss

"Jennifer A. O'Brien masterfully weaves her hard-earned business leadership skills together with her even harder-earned caregiver skills to deliver a comprehensive, practical guide for family caregivers. Learn how to organize your caregiving approach, rally your team, and navigate the healthcare system from someone who has been there, done that, and knows that you can do it too. Family caregivers and healthcare professionals alike would do well to read *Care Boss*."

—**Matthew Tyler**, MD, palliative care physician
and founder of How to Train Your Doctor

"Caregivers are leaders and *Care Boss* shows us how we can do it even better. Jennifer A. O'Brien shares proven techniques from her years of healthcare leadership positions, insights her physician husband imparted, as well as candor and practicality from several intense, sole, family caregiver experiences—making *Care Boss* a not-so-reluctant confession that benefits us all."

—**Natalie Elliott Handy**, founder and chief energy
officer of *Confessions of a Reluctant Caregiver*

"Why do we love this book? Let us count the ways! It is chock-full of practical and tactical tips to help all those caring for others ALSO know how to best care for themselves. And . . . the title. Because caregivers ARE badasses for good, bringing their best selves on the regular—and that makes them a 'care boss.' Thanks for writing your heart to help us in giving ours, Jennifer . . . you are an Archangel extraordinaire in ALL the ways."

—**Alexandra Drane**, CEO and cofounder of Archangels

"*Care Boss* empowers caregivers to be strategic while providing practical, boots-on-the-ground solutions. A new and innovative approach to this commitment of love called caregiving."

—**Brian Bell**, MD, FAAHPM, vice president and chief medical officer of Arkansas Hospice, Inc.

"*Care Boss* is a game changer. Its unique approach—caregiving through the leadership lens—will resonate with healthcare professionals and family caregivers alike."

—**Lisa Pahl**, LCSW, hospice social worker and cocreator of the Death Deck

"An invaluable resource of guidance, inspiration, and empowerment. *Care Boss* is a road map to overcoming challenges, finding balance, and managing the caregiver journey with resilience and strength."

—**Robert Pardi**, leadership coach, founder of Possibility in Action, and eleven-year caregiver for his late wife, Desiree Pardi, MD, PhD

"This heartfelt narrative is a blend of emotional support, practical advice, and actionable strategies to help caregivers navigate the complex and challenging journey of caring for a loved one. *Care Boss* is not just a guide, it's a companion for resilient and dedicated caregivers everywhere. Whether you're a seasoned healthcare professional or new to the role of caregiver, this book offers valuable resources and wisdom."

—***Mike Brown***, former COO of Arkansas Blue Cross Blue Shield

For the family caregivers—the unseen foundation of our society.

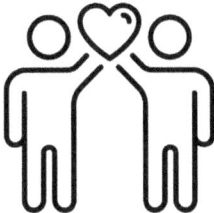

Outline of Contents

Introduction ———————————————————————— 1

- Message: My personal story & why I see you
- Family Caregiving
- Leadership

1. Strategy & Planning ———————————————————— 11

- Message: A story of memories, loss, and looking ahead
- Mission, Vision & Values
- Precious Time
- The Triad of Certainty
- Promises & Future You
- What's Your Mantra?
- Preparing & Planning
- At Peace Tool Kit: A Guide to Being at Peace with End of Life
- To-Do Lists
- Medical Records
- Go Bag

2. Team & Resources ———————————————————— 45

- Message: Feeling entirely alone but not being entirely alone
- Problems with the Word "Team"
- Mapping & Assembling the Helpers
- Family Caregiver Position Description
- Professional Caregivers & Palliative Care
- Advisors
- Family/Circle
- Listening
- Friends & Stakeholders
- Delegation
- Initiating Delegation
- Overcoming Conflict & Obstacles
- Pinpointed Positive Feedback & Thank Yous
- Communication
- Resources
- Social Media

3. Data & Analysis —————————————— 85

- Message: Using my brain to analyze data helps my heart
- Budgeting
- Reporting Periods
- Data-Based Decisions
- Goals
- Treatment Decisions
- Root Cause Analysis
- Urgent/Important Matrix
- The Immeasurable

4. Facility, Environmental Services & Supplies ———— 105

- Message: The shower incident
- Home as Facility
- Medication Management
- Environmental Services (Housekeeping)
- Supplies
- Transport
- Admissions to Professional Facilities

5. Self-Management —————————————— 125

- Message: Never-ending quest
- Water, Food & Rest
- No Self-Care Shaming
- Past, Present & Future Self
- What-Ifs
- Managing the Negative Thought Spiral
- Intensity Assessment Tool
- Emotional Self-Awareness
- Red Phone Friends
- Personal Outlets

6. Beginning to Realize the Vision ——————— 151

- Message: Why didn't the hospice doctor admit himself to hospice sooner?
- Choice, Change & Discharge
- Admission to Hospice & Insurance Coverage
- Duration
- Access & Listen to the Professionals
- DIY
- Medications
- Precious Time
- The Triad of Certainty
- Message: Encouragement

Introduction

New Message

To: Family Caregiver

Subject: My personal story & why I see you . . .

Dear Caregiver,

I have been where you are, and I see you.

More than twenty years ago, my mother's years of chronic illness culminated with a diagnosis of stage IV metastatic pancreatic cancer, and I was her primary caregiver for the five weeks she lived following the diagnosis. About thirteen years later, my beloved husband, Bob, a hospice and palliative care physician, was diagnosed with stage IV metastatic renal clear cell carcinoma. I was his only caregiver for twenty-two months, until he died. Most recently, I was the long-distance caregiver for my father, with whom I had a very strained relationship. Despite the relationship challenges, I was able to provide sound, long-distance caregiving and was with him when he died of heart and lung disease following a hip fracture.

Caregiving for someone you love—or perhaps don't love but have a long-standing relationship with—through a serious, life-limiting condition is both extraordinarily difficult and fulfilling. The statistics indicate that one in five adults in the United States are currently family caregivers,[1] yet there have been few provisions made for us by society, by employers, or even within the health care system. We are, by definition, not financially compensated; as you may know, the other term for "family caregiver" is "uncompensated caregiver," which distinguishes us from professional caregivers (doctors, nurses, etc.), who are paid. Beyond being unpaid, we are often unrecognized; we feel isolated much of the time.

In addition to repeated family caregiver roles, I've worked in the administrative and business aspects of the professional caregiver system for more than thirty-five years. Specifically, I've taught physicians

---
[1] National Alliance for Caregiving (NAC) and AARP, *Caregiving in the US 2020*.

practice management and held numerous management and leadership positions in large practices, academic departments, and health care systems. Most recently, I've been in two consecutive interim chief executive officer (CEO) positions for clinical practices of twenty-five to forty physicians and about two hundred employees.

A CEO certainly enjoys more recognition (for better or for worse) and monetary compensation than a family caregiver, but there are far more similarities to the two roles than differences. Both positions hold tremendous responsibility—and tremendous isolation. Having spent time in both roles in several settings, I've started to think about the similarities, and to realize that family caregivers can benefit from some of the insights and experiences I have as a leader in health care. I've created this guide to help you see and implement the leadership elements of family caregiving.

This book is not meant to be prescriptive, but I hope my observations, experience, and ideas about family caregiving and leadership will give you additional guidance, perspective, and agency as you care for your person. I designed this as a quick read with lots of helpful tips, tricks, and tools, because for family caregivers time is a premium and effectiveness is essential.

My caregiving—with my mother, my husband, and even my father—has been the most important work of my life. With each of their deaths, I transitioned from caregiver to griever. I now carry my experience, memories, and love in a way that helps others.

As I said, I see you. I also understand you, support you, and love you.

—jennifer

Let's start by looking at the basics of both family caregiving and leadership to begin thinking about just how similar they are.

Family Caregiving

AARP (formerly the American Association for Retired Persons) and National Alliance for Caregiving (NAC) conduct an in-depth survey every five years on the topic of family caregiving. The question they ask to identify family caregivers is this:

> **At any time in the last 12 months, has anyone in your household provided unpaid care to a relative or friend 18 years or older to help them care for themselves?** This may include helping with personal needs or household chores. It might be managing a person's finances, arranging for outside services, or visiting regularly to see how they are doing. This adult need not live with you.[2]

You'll notice the definition stipulates that the person may or may not live with you. If you're taking someone to doctor's appointments and visiting them a couple of times a week, that's caregiving. It's also caregiving if you move them in with you or move into their house because they've become unable to live alone. Even if your care recipient lives in a facility such as a nursing home (nearby or far away), you are a family caregiver.

You'll also notice this definition refers to a "relative or friend." You do not have to be caring for a blood relative to be considered a family caregiver. I prefer to use the term "family caregiver" because "uncompensated," while true, seems cold and depressing. The terms "caretaker," "carer," "care companion," and "care partner" are used as well. I use the term "family caregiver" throughout this book because it denotes the giving and uncompensated nature of the

---

[2] National Alliance for Caregiving (NAC) and AARP, *Caregiving in the US 2020*.

position, and because it distinguishes us from professional caregivers such as physicians and nurses.

So, if your answer to the question above is "yes," it means you are a family caregiver. You might initially shrug at that and say, "I am *just* the daughter." Or "It's my duty as a daughter/spouse/son/friend." Perhaps because you are the daughter, son, spouse, or grandchild, you think it is just expected. Or maybe you know that no one will do it if you don't. Either or both may be true. Regardless, you are, by definition, a family caregiver, and there is no more important and serious job and set of responsibilities on this planet.

Leadership

Based on my experience as a manager, director, and chief executive officer (and based on what I've observed in other leaders), I offer that leadership, in a nutshell, comes down to three functions:

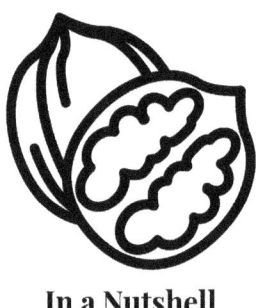

In a Nutshell

- Setting the vision
- Bringing everything together
- Communicating effectively

When these three functions come together consistently and successfully—and when inspiration is present—effective leadership is happening.

Like caregiving, leadership is lonely and weighty. An enlightening study found that half of CEOs feel lonely and isolated, and of those, 61 percent feel that isolation and loneliness impact their performance adversely.[3] When I am in a CEO position, I feel an underlying isolation. I see it as my job to give credit to the team or other individuals for successes, and to take responsibility for the failures. There is a profound loneliness in that. A CEO has a layer and level of burden that, organizationally, no one else quite has.

As a CEO, I feel I must make my own joy. For example, as I credit a group or individual for an accomplishment, I tell myself that my leadership provided the environment and support that helped them to succeed for the organization.

Also, as CEO, I feel responsible for the hundreds of employees and even more patients and family members on the premises each day. My most recent CEO position had about two hundred employees, and we did one thousand patient encounters on most weekdays. Each day I felt the responsibility of those as "souls on board," somewhat like I imagine a commercial airline pilot does.

In another survey, 68 percent of leaders admitted they were not fully prepared for the job.[4] Lonely, isolated, pressured, and ill-prepared. Hmmm . . . sounds just like the predominant feelings of a family caregiver to me. What do you think?

---

[3] Thomas J. Saparito, "It's Time to Acknowledge CEO Loneliness," *Harvard Business Review* (February 2012).
[4] Kati Najipoor-Schutte and Dick Patton, "Survey: 68% of CEOs Admit They Weren't Fully Prepared for the Job," *Harvard Business Review* (July 2018).

So, we have acknowledged similarities in the challenges of both caregiving and leadership. Now, let's look at reframing those challenges. Fortunately for caregivers, the similarities aren't limited to the realm of challenges. Many of the same qualities, values, and skills that make for great leadership can also support your caregiving. Family caregivers may not all have specialized training or certification, but we can all draw on what we've learned from other leadership experiences to be effective caregivers.

The words below are associated with both leadership and family caregiving. Start your thought process and contribution by adding some terms to the clipboard below.

- authenticity
- balance
- commitment
- common sense
- communication
- compassion
- confidence
- courage
- delegation
- determination
- empowerment
- energy
- experience
- focus
- genuineness
- honesty
- humility
- integrity
- intuition
- listening ability
- openness
- people focus
- principles
- purpose
- reason
- risk
- sensitivity
- sincerity
- strategy
- values

Add some others

☐ Resilience
☐ Adaptability
☐ _____
☐ _____
☐ _____
☐ _____
☐ _____

Rather than Chief *Executive* Officer, "CEO," in caregiving it is more accurately defined as Chief *Everything* Officer. This is because in addition to setting the vision, bringing everything together, and communicating effectively, caregivers are called upon to get deep into the minutiae and the day-to-day as subject matter experts and front line workers.

In the next six sections—Strategy & Planning; Team & Resources; Data & Analysis; Facility, Environmental Services & Supplies; Self-Management; and Beginning to Realize the Vision—I'll share my health care leadership and family caregiving experiences, along with a few personal stories, in hopes of empowering you with the perspective and resources to carry out your caregiving as Chief Everything Officer, comprehensive leadership position that it is.

1

Strategy & Planning

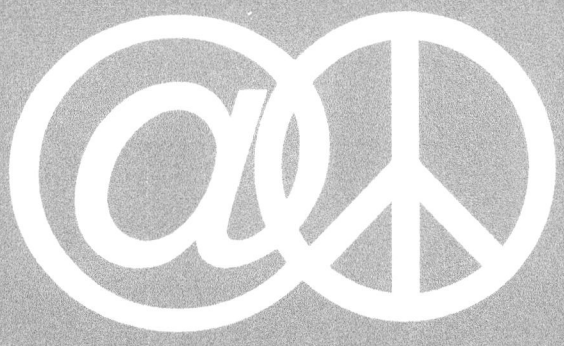

New Message

To: Family Caregiver

Subject: A story of memories, loss, and looking ahead

Dear Caregiver,

In 1983, September 29 was a Thursday. I was in the third week of my freshman year away at college. It may have been the first day since leaving home that I felt adjusted and had woken up, dressed, and gone to breakfast and then to class without the lump of homesickness in my throat.

The day was so clear and beautiful. I walked the considerable distance back to my dorm after morning classes. I was wearing a colorful Esprit skirt and a purple, boxy sweater. As I entered my room, the large black rotary phone that swiveled between two dorm rooms was ringing. I answered the phone, and a man's voice came on and said, "Jennifer, this is Mr. Sherman, Keith's dad." Before I had time to register my confusion about why the father of a boy in my younger brother's class was phoning me in my college dorm room, he said, "I'd like you to sit down, please." The news is never good when they insist you sit before the telling.

Keith's dad told me my thirteen-year-old brother, David, had been in an accident. He was still alive, in a coma, and Mr. Sherman had arranged the three connecting flights for me to return home.

I went home, and each day we focused on what was immediately in front of us. We coated David's lips with balm, because they were chapping from the ventilator mouthpiece. We applied tape, sometimes, to keep his eyelids shut so that his eyes didn't dry out from being partially open. We waited for lab and brain imaging results every few days.

Exactly three weeks after the accident, when images showed

his brain activity had dwindled to nothing, my parents made the heart-wrenching decision to extubate him, and he was pronounced dead on October 20, 1983.

David was my only sibling. At age eighteen the Universe taught me in no uncertain terms that at the end of life comes death. I learned there is no dress rehearsal or do-over for the death of a loved one. And as the years went on, his death, as much as—perhaps more than—his life, stayed with me, shaped me, and became a part of my life.

I share this story as an introduction to the Strategy & Planning section because, in addition to the day-to-day, effective caregivers must consider the big picture. That is, while much of the material here is also applicable to caring for a family member who will recover, for the most part, this book is specific to a care recipient who has a serious, life-limiting condition and who will likely precede the family caregiver in death.

Simply put, it is impossible to effectively plan and look ahead without addressing *all* aspects of the future, including not just tomorrow's to-do list but the disease or condition's progression, the death of your care recipient, your subsequent transition from caregiver to griever, and your life after caregiving.

Nothing about this is easy. But then, you know that. By looking at family caregiving through the leadership lens, I hope you will feel empowered to be proactive about what is ahead with your care recipient, as well as about what comes later, when you go on without them.

I have been where you are. I see you, I understand you, and I know you can do this.

—jennifer

One November afternoon a little over a year before he died, my husband, Bob, and I sat before the notary public to transfer the cars and other property to my name in preparation for his death and my survivorship. The notary asked why we were transferring ownership and I responded, "Because Bob is dying."

She became visibly nervous and distracted, so I said, "We're at peace with it." I had heard Bob say this many times, and for the most part it was true. That evening, I created the design on page 11 about being at peace with end of life and put it in the art journal I was keeping.

I have chosen to use this image as the symbol for the Strategy & Planning section of this book because forethought and planning are essential to finding peace in caregiving and at the end of life.

The contents of this section:

- Mission, Vision & Values
    - Develop the Mission Statement
    - Develop the Vision Statement
    - Mission & Vision Statements for Your Use
    - Identify & Document Core Values
    - Post the Mission, Vision & Values
- Precious Time
- The Triad of Certainty
- Promises & Future You
- What's Your Mantra?
- Preparing & Planning
- At Peace Tool Kit: A Guide to Being at Peace with End of Life
    - Set Up Smartphone Medical ID
    - Set Up Smartphone Legacy Contacts
    - Establish Advance Health Care Directives and Proxies
    - Administrative Details
- To-Do Lists
- Medical Records
- Go Bag

Mission, Vision & Values

Strategy and planning must begin with mission, vision, and values. If you have ever wondered about these terms, what they really mean, and why they are important, you are not alone. They may seem a bit opaque and ethereal for a busy family caregiver, but they are super important in leadership and in seeing the big picture. After all, we said leadership is setting the vision, bringing everything together, and communicating effectively. Mission, vision, and values are a big part of all three of those, so let's define them here:

- The *mission* is a concise statement of purpose, reason for existence, and ongoing objectives. The mission is what we *do*.
- The *vision* is an equally concise description of aspirations, goals, and the future. The vision is what we hope to *become*.
- The *values* are our core ethics, morals, principles, and beliefs. They guide our decisions, actions, and conduct as we carry out the mission and progress toward the vision. The values are the *why* and the *way* we do what we do.

Develop the Mission Statement

To develop the mission for your family caregiving situation, ask and answer these questions:

- What do I do?
- What is my purpose?
- What are my overall objectives?

Take some time with these questions. You may not be able to make a complete list in one sitting—that's okay; in fact, it is preferred. These are big questions with many answers that deserve some time and thought. In the space below, write the single words and phrases that come to mind as you answer the three questions above:

Next, highlight the words and phrases that stand out as most important. Eliminate or consolidate redundancies. Consider all of the words and phrases carefully and put together a few sentences to create a concise mission statement:

Develop the Vision Statement

To write the vision statement—your future aspirations for yourself as a family caregiver and beyond—ask and answer the questions:

- What does the ideal progression look like for my care recipient?
- What do I want my future, near and distant, to be?
- What does success in this situation mean for me, the family caregiver?

Here again, take some time with these questions. Write the single words and phrases that come to mind:

Next, highlight the words and phrases that stand out as most important. Eliminate or consolidate redundancies. Consider all of the words and phrases carefully and put together a few sentences to create a concise vision statement:

Note: Even though it may be hard and painful to think about the end of your care recipient's life, only by considering what that looks like—and how you go on afterward—can you fully explore and develop a vision for your caregiving.

Mission & Vision Statements for Your Use

I did the mission and vision development exercises again recently, with the benefit of my own family caregiving experiences, hindsight, and several years now of advocating for family caregivers. These are the statements I came up with; you are welcome to incorporate them into your own or use them as is.

Mission

Ensure safety, nourishment, hygiene, companionship, advocacy, access, agency, and care for my care recipient, while seeing him for the person he is and not trying to change or fix him.

Vision

A comfortable, dignified end of life for my care recipient; a smooth transition from caregiver to griever; and an emotionally, mentally, spiritually, and physically healthy future for me.

In a journal entry that became part of my book *The Hospice Doctor's Widow: An Art Journal of Caregiving and Grief*, I wrote, "We are going through two different processes. He is dying. I am surviving."

Those two processes were thoroughly intertwined, yet my husband and I were headed toward two different futures. I had to proactively consider how I would likely feel and live in the future after his death. We will address much more on family caregiver well-being in the Self-Management section.

Identify & Document Core Values

Values are our core ethics, morals, principles, and beliefs. They guide our decisions, actions, and conduct as we carry out the mission and navigate toward the vision. The values are the *why* and the *way* we do what we do.

Values are our core. We believe in them; we follow them; we preserve them, practice them, and stand up for them. Determining the core values of the caregiving situation may be a bit different from determining those of an organization, because there are two (or more) *individuals* rather than an organization that is made up of many people and parts. Additionally, the caregiving situation is emotionally charged and involves the essence of life and, ultimately, death.

Thus, it is essential to explore and document your own values as the caregiver as well as those of your care recipient. If there are others in the inner circle, perhaps your care recipient's siblings or spouse, their values must be considered as well.

Complete the following exercise to state the most and least important values you each hold. In the spaces in the third column, list those that are on both of your lists. As you consider what to include, focus on values that relate to caregiving and end-of-life situations such as:

- being as comfortable as possible (or not)
- living as independently as possible (or not)
- letting things happen naturally (or not)
- being able to spend time and leave memories with friends and family (or not)
- lingering (or not)
- utilizing every possible life-extending measure (or not)
- staying true to faith, religion, or beliefs (or not)
- contributing to clinical science efforts (or not)
- avoiding expensive care (or not)
- and so on.

If, because of cognitive or other impairment, you, the caregiver, are completing the care recipient's lists for them, do your best to draw on your historical knowledge, your objectivity, and perhaps the input of others to create a list that truly reflects your care recipient's values.

If there are one or more other stakeholders in the situation, add columns as needed, and engage each person in this process.

Shared values unite people and drive decisions, innovations, and problem-solving. Identifying shared values will be key to your caregiver-as-leader efficacy. For example, my late husband, Bob, and I both valued thorough preparation for end of life. We both worked hard to prepare for his death and my survivorship.

You may discover significant differences in core values. A value that your care recipient lists as most important may be among your least important. Identifying differences is as important as identifying values that are shared.

In my father's old age, he developed ideological views very different from what he had held for most of his life—and from my own views. It was important to recognize those differences so that we could respect each other and agree to disagree. As his health care proxy and caregiver, it was essential that I represent what *he* wanted for *his* care and end of life, even if it was different from what I would want for myself, or from my wishes for him. So consider any items on each of the "most important" lists that are *not* shared, and list them in the bottom section.

Identifying shared values will help when it's time to build consensus and make decisions together. Noting where your values differ will help you deliberately and respectfully navigate the changes and decisions that the caregiving situation presents as it progresses.

Caregiver	Care Recipient	Shared
Most important values:	Most important values:	Most important values that are shared:
Least important values:	Least important values:	Least important values that are shared:

Highlight or note here differences that need to be respected and considered.

Post the Mission, Vision & Values

The mission, vision, and values are at the very core of effective leadership. Once you have established them, document them in a clear way and put them in a place or places where you will see them with some frequency. They are not the Magna Carta; if you discover along the way that you left something out, add it. If something needs to be reworded or changed, do it.

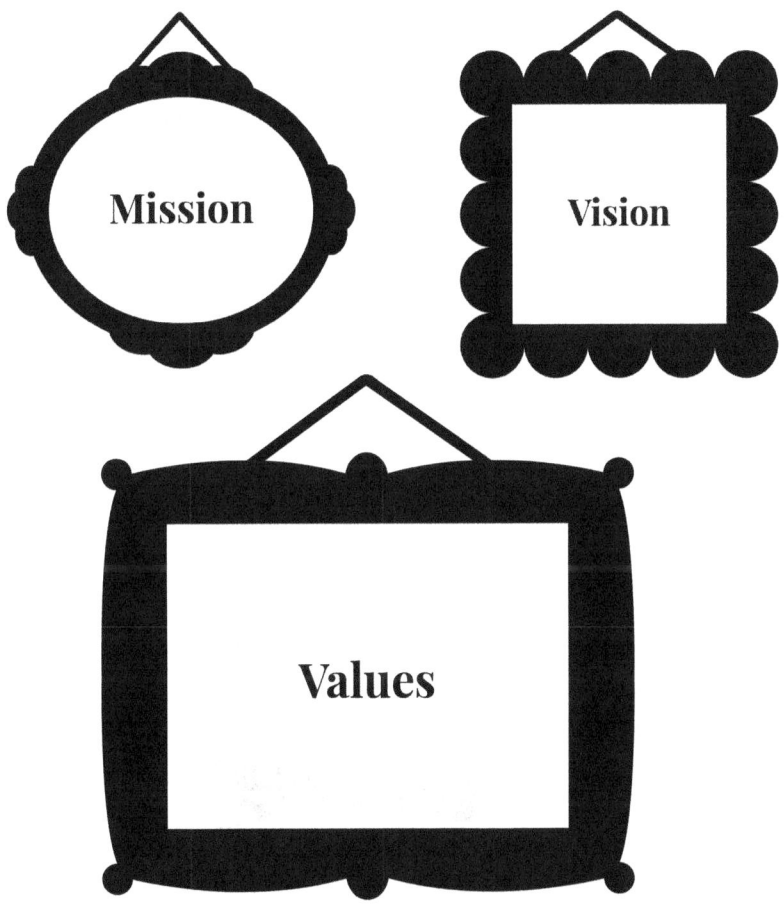

Precious Time

On the topic of mission and vision for family caregiving, it seems only appropriate to share the concept of Precious Time.

The term was coined by my late husband, Bob Lehmberg, MD, a palliative care physician, who would tell patients and families, "You are into *Precious* Time," to help them understand that death was nearing. Precious Time doesn't so much mean that time is precious (although it certainly is). Instead, *Precious* Time, with emphasis on the first word, is a type of time.

Precious Time is when death is imminent. Precious Time is when you lean in further and make your love and care known, because this person will soon die, and then you will go on living. There is no dress rehearsal for the death of your care recipient. When you enter Precious Time with your care recipient, the vision starts to be realized. You will not get a do-over. This may be one of the biggest events of your life. You will carry it and how you managed it for the rest of your life. The final section of this book, Beginning to Realize the Vision, goes into more depth and detail about the time when death is nearing.

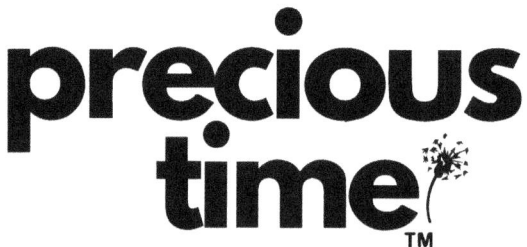

The Triad of Certainty

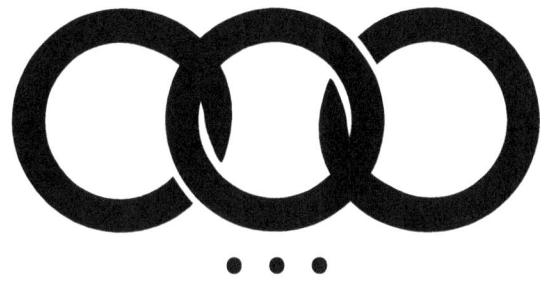

The Triad of Certainty

At the end of life comes death.
There are no do-overs in end of life.
Changed forever, loved ones remain and remember.

Promises & Future You

Hope is not a strategy.

—Vince Lombardi

Effective CEOs may set and achieve ambitious goals, but they do not commit to accomplishing the impossible or make promises they may not be able to keep. The family caregiver job is huge and already feels impossible. Please do not add to your future burden by making promises that may not be within your ability to keep.

Do not promise your care recipient:

- you will never admit them to a care facility.
- they will die at home.
- you will always be there.

Stay away from the words "always" and "never" when discussing the future. These words are too extreme and indicate declarations that may not be within your power to carry out.

Think of your future self.

In response to this you might think, "Well, my care recipient has advanced dementia, so they won't remember if I make a promise and am not able to keep it." But here's the thing: You will remember that you made a promise and did not keep it. And right there you may have jeopardized a portion of the vision—your future emotional and mental health.

If your care recipient tries to get you to commit to a broad declaration, say, "I understand that is a priority. *Together*, we will do everything in *our* power to _____, but I cannot commit to that as a promise." With this phrasing, you are acknowledging to your care recipient that you understand their desire and goal. By using "we," you are including their participation rather than putting all the responsibility on yourself. Again, if your care recipient does not have the cognitive ability to understand, you are doing this for the health and well-being of your future self.

What's Your Mantra?

A mantra uses simple language so that everyone understands. It can be posted, repeated, and said in unison with others who might need reminding.

Create a mantra that grounds you, and post it in places where you will see it frequently. Repeat it to yourself and others when necessary. As CEO of several different health care organizations, I took this management mantra with me:

*Work hard, work smart, **and** be kind.*

I shared this mantra with managers. It provided a baseline when evaluating an employee or an incident. The "and" is important, because all three parts of the mantra are of equal importance. That is, just because someone is an excellent nurse does not mean we ignore the nurse's inability to be kind to other employees.

During his illness, Bob had this mantra:

In acceptance lies peace.

Feeling at peace was very important to Bob. It was to me as well, yet as his only caregiver I probably came back just as much to these words:

We're going through two different processes—he is dying; I am surviving.

This mantra also served me well:

Hope for the best and prepare for the worst.

As a family caregiver, balancing two seemingly different or even opposite notions with "and" rather than "or" or "but" is important. An easy-to-repeat phrase that contains such contrast can help you move through the day-to-day of the mission and toward the successful realization of the vision.

I wrote another mantra of sorts at the end of my last couple of updates to friends and family as Bob was dying. I repeated it to myself in the last few days of his life:

The miracle is peace.

This mantra kept the notion of a quick, quiet, and comfortable death at our center.

Preparing & Planning

By failing to prepare,
you are preparing to fail.

—Benjamin Franklin

Realizing an ambitious vision such as a comfortable, dignified death, a smooth transition from caregiver to griever, and a healthy future won't happen by mantra alone. The successful realization of this trifold vision will begin with planning, preparation, discussions, and decisions.

When my mother was diagnosed with cancer, we almost immediately drew up an agreement for her to sell me her car for $1, and we talked about her specific requests for the disposition of her remains and her memorial service. (And boy were they specific: She wanted me to have her cremated, host her memorial service no less than six weeks after her death so that people flying in could get a less expensive airfare, and hire a New Orleans–style brass band to play "When the Saints Go Marching In.") We also got a lot of administrative preparation done in the five weeks she lived following the diagnosis.

With my late husband, it was similar, although we made far more and larger preparations for his death and my survivorship. We revisited his already-complete, comprehensive, end-of-life documents to be sure I felt comfortable carrying out his wishes if he became unable to speak for himself. We downsized our life, sold our house, and moved into a condominium that he knew I would feel more comfortable in by myself. As I've mentioned, we put all the property and cars in my name. He gave me specifics on what he wanted for his remains disposition and memorial service.

None of this preparation made me any less sad when they died. It did, however, help me feel less lost and confused in the days and hours before their deaths, as well as in the weeks, months, even years after. My transition from caregiver to griever was unencumbered by the exhaustive details, time-consuming tasks, and higher costs of an ill-prepared-for death.

A recent study shows the average time it takes survivors to settle matters following a death is fifteen months.[5] I can tell you I spent nowhere near that much time following any of my loved ones' deaths, because they were all so well prepared.

Comprehensive end-of-life preparation and planning is not unlike the effort put into bringing a pregnancy to term with a healthy delivery. A pregnant person typically has eighteen to twenty visits with an obstetrician or midwife to prepare. And while they do not know if the delivery will call for episiotomy, epidural, or Cesarean section, all those possibilities are thoroughly discussed and considered well in advance. Consider putting just as much deliberation, planning, and preparation into end of life.

The following tool kit will take you through the key elements of planning and preparation. By completing it, you'll prepare for the future just as a leader develops pro forma documents and projections. Expect this to take some time; a realistic timeline for completing the tool kit may be as long as several weeks or a few months. Consider completing one tool kit for your care recipient and one for yourself.

---

[5] Empathy, "The Cost of Dying" (2024).

At Peace Tool Kit: A Guide to Being at Peace with End of Life

1. Set Up Smartphone Medical ID

If your care recipient carries a smartphone or tablet, set up the Medical ID feature and list all the essential information. This is easy and quick. Do it right now so that if there is a medical emergency, responders can access key information and emergency contacts from the device. The iPhone has a built-in Medical ID feature. Many other devices do not; however, there are Medical ID apps available. After loading the information, change the settings so that the information can be accessed even when the device is locked. Do this on your care recipient's device and your own device, share the information with others in your family or circle, and insist they do the same. Emergency health care professionals can be more effective in caring for patients if this information is readily available.

2. Set Up Smartphone Legacy Contacts

Individuals who are designated as legacy contacts on devices and accounts will be given access upon the death of the account holder. If you do not have full access to your care recipient's devices, set up legacy contacts for the devices/accounts as soon as possible.

I am in several social media groups that support widowed people, and a couple of times each week a newly widowed person shares that their person died without designating a legacy contact or sharing their password or personal identification access. That widowed person has lost access to all the photos, videos, and contacts that, with the death of the individual, have become more important than ever. Carriers and device companies will not simply give you access to a deceased person's account and data unless you are a designated legacy contact. Each time an incorrect "guess" is entered in an attempt to get in, the device gets closer to being deactivated forever.

On Apple devices, legacy contacts can be set up within the security settings. For all other devices, seek out the instructions for legacy contact assignments and make them as soon as possible. You will also want to set up legacy contacts for any social media accounts.

3. Establish Advance Health Care Directives & Proxies

Every adult has the right and responsibility to document and communicate advance health care directives / advance care planning, and to designate a health care proxy / medical representative. A health care proxy is the adult you have shared your health care and end-of-life wishes with and designated to speak for you and make medical decisions on your behalf if you are unable to do so yourself. Designate an alternate health care proxy just in case your primary one is unable to serve in that capacity at the needed time.

A family caregiver is not a de facto health care proxy. For example, if a parent knows that one adult child will likely be their caregiver but feels that person may have difficulty representing health care wishes and intentions when the time comes, they may designate another adult child as the proxy.

The specifics of creating these plans vary by region, but most states and provinces have public guidelines and forms that allow individuals to establish and document their advance health care directives without a doctor or attorney. To find the information for your state or province, visit CaringInfo.org/Planning/Advance-Directives (United States) or AdvanceCarePlanning.ca (Canada), or search "advance health care directives" and the name of your state or province.

Most health insurance plans cover one or more physician visits for guidance in establishing advance health care directives, and most attorneys who do estate planning include documenting advance health care directives and proxies as part of their menu of services.

When the advance directive and proxy documents have been finalized, make sure that copies are distributed to your care recipient's physicians, as well as to the proxy and alternate proxy. Put a copy of the documents in the file or notebook where you keep other essential health care information for your care recipient. Keep a wallet card and/or note in your care recipient's device's Medical ID to indicate that they have documented advance directives. Advance directives in their entirety are not stored in the Medical ID of a device.

If your care recipient's advance directives include a Do Not Resuscitate (DNR) document, also known as an Allow Natural Death (AND) or a Physician/Medical Orders for Life-Sustaining Treatment (POLST or MOLST), or any additional advance directives, affix copies of all of them to the refrigerator in the kitchen, and always leave them there. The kitchen refrigerator is the only place that emergency medical technicians (EMTs) will look for these important documents.

4. Administrative Details

Each year money, property, and precious items such as digital photos get lost or left behind because people die without organizing and communicating. These losses only add to the sadness of the death. Consider the vision. Death is one of the few certainties in life. Your care recipient is likely to die before you do. The loss of important documents, photos, and special keepsakes is entirely avoidable with just a little bit of forethought and effort. Please use the following prompts to gather assets, store them, and make them accessible to ease the after-loss burden.

Securely document the access codes to all phones, tablets, laptops, desktop computers, etc. using a password management system. There are several password management systems available, including NordPass, Keeper, RoboForm, Norton Password Manager, 1Password, etc. Smartphones also include password tracking systems for passwords you enter while using the phone. Research what works best for you.

Social media accounts left unattended after a death can open surviving loved ones up to scams, fraud, and other ugly behavior.

Some platforms, such as Facebook, have a remembrance feature that allows the account to remain, managed by a legacy contact, with a designation that the account's original holder is deceased. As mentioned in the earlier discussion of legacy contacts, make sure to designate legacy wishes on all social media pages and other communication platforms.

Next, gather the details and documentation for each of the following:

Financial Accounts

- Checking
    - Bank Name:
    - Name on Account:
    - Account Number:
- Savings
    - Bank Name:
    - Name on Account:
    - Account Number:
- 401(k) / IRA / Retirement Account(s)
    - Institution Name:
    - Name on Account:
    - Account Number:
- Investment(s)
    - Institution Name:
    - Name on Account:
    - Account Number:
- Cryptocurrency/NFTs
- Other Digital Assets

Legal Documents

- Complete or gather the following. Store in a fireproof lockbox.
    - Attorney(s) name(s) and contact information
    - Trust document(s)
    - Last will and testament
    - Power of attorney (financial and property)

- Power of attorney (health care—null and void once the person dies)
- Permissions re: use of likeness, voice, and image in the creation of digital resurrection/restoration
- Other
- Titles, Deeds, and Certificates
    - Birth certificate
    - Marriage certificate
    - Divorce papers
    - Passport
    - Home title
    - Land title
    - Automobile title(s)
    - Recreational vehicle title(s)
    - Stock and bond documentation
    - Copyrights, patents, and other intellectual property documents
    - Firearm documentation
    - Cemetery deed
- Insurance Policies
    - Health
    - Employer life
    - Individual life
    - Long-term disability
    - Disability / serious illness
    - Annuity documentation
    - Auto
    - Umbrella
    - Homeowners
    - Burial
    - Other
- Additional Important Information and Documents
    - Documents related to dependents and pets
    - Storage facility rental and access information
    - Safe deposit box documentation and key
    - List of items to be gifted and recipients

- Special instructions
- Letters and upon-death correspondence
- Documentation of loans and debts owed to estate
- List of key contacts
- Disposition, memorial, and obituary instructions

As thorough as this tool kit is, it may not be enough to get the job done. Just as leaders hire coaches and advisors to be more effective and accountable in completing big, important tasks, family caregivers can also be assisted by hiring an end-of-life planning coach, advisor, or doula. These firms and individuals are experts regarding specific resources and can deal with all of the issues, including the emotional, familial, and cultural. More on advisors in the Team & Resources section.

To-Do Lists

Few planning practices have helped me more, in both CEOing and family caregiving, than my daily to-do list method. Here are my five top tips for more effective to-do lists:

1. Your modality of choice is best.

The "best" technology is only effective if it's used consistently. So, for me, a pocket notebook is more effective than an app. I carry a notebook about the same size as my phone. I use it all day, every day, and it consistently helps me complete my tasks and overall goals. If an app (e.g., Notion or Asana) works for you, use it. If you prefer a larger notebook, use that. Use what works for you.

2. Ambitious realism.

Be determined with your daily list, but only include tasks you can realistically complete. An overly zealous list will generate a sense of defeat before you even get started, and a to-do list full of simple actions you take automatically will become cluttered and easy to ignore. So it's best to mainly list tasks that are difficult but possible. Do include basic tasks such as showering or working out if they are feeling particularly challenging, and consider changing them up a little. For example, instead of "Shower" and "Exercise," write, "Listen to a podcast in the shower" or "Skip the treadmill; walk in the park." This pairing or reframing may make them more attractive and provide incentive.

3. Just me and the Universe.

Each page of my mini notebook says "Me" at the top left, the day's date in the middle, and "Universe" at the top right. If you prefer alternative terms such as "Tasks" and "Goals," use your own language. My daily "Me" list includes individual items I need to get done in a timely manner. My "Universe" list includes larger projects

I need to keep in mind that are unlikely to get done today or even tomorrow. This list includes upcoming deadlines and big stuff requiring more help or attention.

4. Get help from the Universe.

The Universe list represents:

- Larger projects to keep in mind
- Upcoming deadlines
- Big stuff that may require help from others or a larger force.

The first two items above (about larger projects and deadlines) help me with the concrete actions I need to take or prepare for. The third point refers to the "big stuff." I learned the power of listing the "big stuff" while caregiving for my husband. I started to list the positive actions, effects, or results I wanted the Universe to provide, rather than worrying about all the possible bad or suboptimal happenings. For several years now I have been replacing my worries with positive directives for the Universe. Basically, I have been replacing my what-if fears with corresponding what-if hopes, and it has helped me tremendously. There's more on what-ifs in the Self-Management section.

5. Mark completed tasks as done.

This is important for two reasons: to celebrate an accomplishment and to see what needs to be done next. I prefer one or two thin lines through the task rather than completely redacting it. This way, I can still read the task if I need to look back at some point. You can also draw a little box or line next to each item to color or make a check mark in it upon completion. Again, do what works best for you.

On the following page are two daily lists. The first includes examples from a typical day in a CEO position. The second is from a day in my life when I was my beloved Bob's caregiver. Closer to the end of Bob's life, my Universe list included that he would live through the holidays and would die quickly and quietly when the time came. (Both happened.)

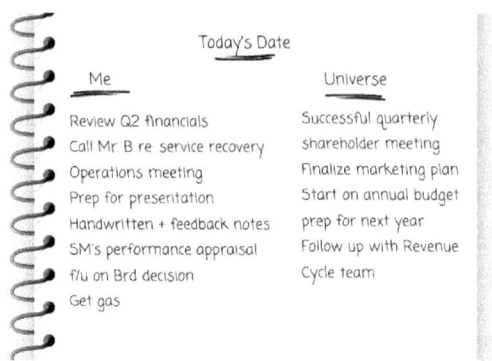

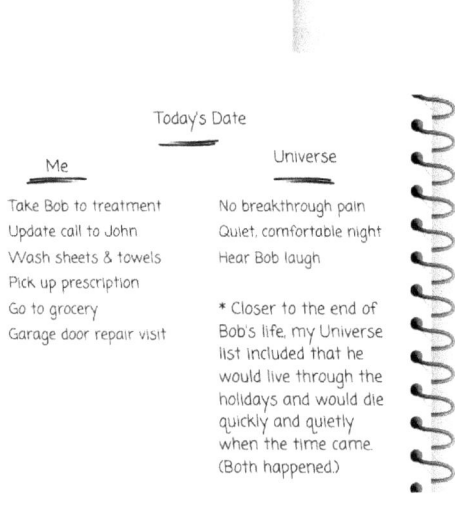

Medical Records

Medical Records

As advanced as some health care technologies have become, electronic medical records systems are not interconnected between various facilities and locations. To be prepared for each and every planned visit and service as well as the emergent ones, put together a file, envelope, or sleeve that you can easily grab and take with you when your care recipient has a health care appointment or an emergency. This portable record should include the following details for the care recipient:

- Full name
- Date of birth
- Address
- All known allergies
- Current medications list: Include reason, dose, and frequency.
- List of physicians: Include contact information, specialty, and what they are treating.
- List of diagnoses and medical conditions
- Emergency contact(s): For each, include full name, relationship, and cell phone number.
- Health care proxy and alternate health care proxy: Include full names and contact information.
- Signed HIPAA release for anyone with whom medical professionals may need to discuss private health care information
- Advance directives
- Durable power of attorney
- Health insurance coverage details
- Do Not Resuscitate (DNR) / Allow Natural Death (AND) documents
- Physician/Medical Orders for Life-Sustaining Treatment (POLST/MOLST), if applicable

- Blank paper or notebook for notetaking during visits and conversations with health care professionals
- Any other legal documentation that is appropriate, helpful, or necessary

If a paper file will not work because of portability between family caregivers, scan these documents and create a secure pdf file on your smartphone or other device.

Go Bag

As I mentioned in my first message to you, I was the long-distance family caregiver to my father, who had severe heart and lung disease for many years before he died. He lived a forty-five-minute drive from the nearest small community hospital and up to a two-and-a-half-hour drive from more specialized hospitals and physician practices. The paid caregiver who drove him to doctor visits or the emergency department would inevitably fail to bring key items along. The caregiver would get my dad to the hospital (he often had to be admitted because of breathing problems) and would then need to turn around and make the same drive to get items such as my dad's phone charger, glasses, toiletries, personal items, etc. This was a waste of time and resources.

Think about the overnight bag that Nancy Drew kept in the trunk of her car or the labor and delivery bag that an expectant mother keeps readily available in the last weeks of her pregnancy. Create a bag with an extra charger, a pair of readers, and any other basics. Take the go bag with you anytime you must travel long distances for doctor's appointments or other health care, because sometimes those outpatient services turn into hospital admissions.

2

Team & Resources

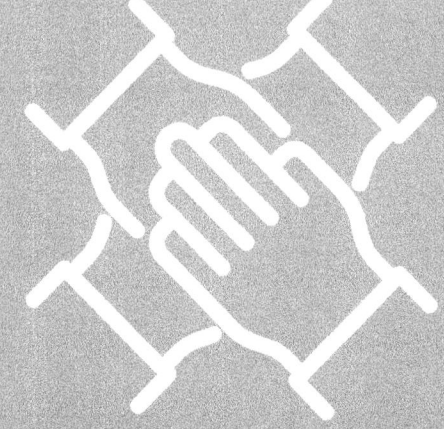

New Message

To: Family Caregiver

Subject: Feeling entirely alone but not being entirely alone

Dear Caregiver,

When my mother was diagnosed with terminal cancer, her mother was still alive. My mother had been living with my grandmother as a care companion. Immediately, I moved in with my grandmother and took over with her, because my mother had to be in a facility. My mother was the oldest of seven. So, while I did have responsibility for my grandmother, several of my mom's siblings were a huge help taking shifts at the hospice facility and taking delegation direction when I offered it. Still, it was my mom who was dying, my only sibling had died many years earlier, and I *felt* very alone.

My husband was a different story. Neither of us had any family in town. Because he was a well-known physician in our small town, he felt strongly about maintaining his privacy and about us taking care of everything without help from others. I totally understood this, would have felt the same way if it were me, and wanted nothing more than to honor his wishes. Still, there were people who came through for us. A friend would periodically and reliably take me out for a coffee and just listen and let me vent without any judgment. Two physician friends of Bob's were very good about checking in on him and taking him out and on short trips when he was able. And, of course, we had his oncologist and pain management physician, who were very responsive whenever Bob needed anything. Still, I felt very alone, and my husband was dying, which would soon leave me unequivocally alone.

My father managed to become a grumpy recluse in the last twenty-five years of his life. He and my mother had divorced about five years before my brother died. He had never remarried (neither of them did). He lived in a very rural setting, became a bit of a hoarder, and did not practice personal hygiene. He did not have any friends, and the people he had contact with were those I had hired to try to clean things up around his place and take him grocery shopping and to doctor's appointments. I was long-distance, and I was indeed very alone. When he broke his hip and was nearing death, an old friend of our family's was extremely helpful to me, letting me stay with her for two weeks and offering all sorts of help when I traveled out to be with him as he died in a hospital setting.

What I am trying to share here is that as a family caregiver I have always *felt* alone. Caregiving for someone you love who will (likely) precede you in death is lonely. And, if you are anything like me, the lonelier it feels the more determined you become to do it all—and do it all by yourself. Do not fall prey to this self-determination.

You are not alone. You have me. You have this book, where I am trying to share everything I know that might help you. And there *are* others. Some may see you and understand; others won't, but they can still help. Sometimes I think one of the most difficult aspects of family caregiving is recognizing the opportunity to accept or ask for help, and then doing it.

I have been where you are. You are not alone. I see you, I understand you, and I know you can do this.

—jennifer

Don't say "team" when you mean "me."

By now, we have made several strong correlations between the role of a CEO and that of a family caregiver. As we introduce this new section, Team & Resources, you might let out a sarcastic chuckle when you read the word "team." As a family caregiver, especially if you are the sole caregiver, it can feel as though you are a team of one. Having said that, let's explore the other people in the story of you and your care recipient. There are others.

There are physicians and other professional caregivers. There may be family members. There are friends. There are advisors. There are volunteers from organizations. There really are others.

The contents of this section:

- Problems with the Word "Team"
- Mapping & Assembling the Helpers
    - Make a List of Those Who Do Help
    - Make a List of Those Who Can Help
- Organizational Chart
- Family Caregiver Position Description
- Professional Caregivers & Palliative Care
- Advisors
- Family/Circle
    - Meetings & Communication
    - Sample Family/Circle Meeting Agenda
- Listening
- Friends & Stakeholders
- Delegation
- Initiating Delegation
    - Determine Tasks & Responsibilities to Delegate
    - Identify Who Is Best for Each Task
    - Communicate Clearly, Including Deadlines
- Overcoming Conflict & Obstacles
- Pinpointed Positive Feedback & Thank Yous
- Communication
- Resources
- Social Media

Problems with the Word "Team"

Let's consider the word "team." It frequently leaves one thinking about basketball or football. This all leads to cheering, empty hype, and words like "winning" and "scoring." Well-meaning visitors use sports analogies incorrectly or take them too far, saying stuff like, "We're all on the same team— you're the quarterback." Meanwhile you the caregiver are wondering, "Where are the *receivers* to catch the ball when I am about to be sacked?"

The word "team" is often used euphemistically when the more accurate term is "group." If visitors and relatives who are more removed from the day-to-day caregiving insist on using sports and team terms, you could let them know that it feels more like you are on your own doing an Ironman triathlon. If you take this approach, be ready with answers or plan to follow up when they say, "What can I do to help?"

Another option is to redirect them to the notion of a ski or gymnastics team, where each individual contributes their own top performance one at a time so that team success can be achieved. This type of reframing is part of the facilitation and communication necessary to identify who is in the group or on the team and inspire them to be their best and contribute positively.

Mapping & Assembling the Helpers

The first step to identifying helpers is to make some lists. Think about those who have already started helping, those who have offered, and those who could and would help if asked.

Make a List of Those Who Do Help

As primary family caregiver, think about the other care helpers involved. Who are they? List them.

_____   _____

_____   _____

_____   _____

_____   _____

_____   _____

_____   _____

Make a List of Those Who Can Help

Now, think about those who have offered help but you have declined or deferred—and those who probably could help (or help more). Who are they? List them.

_____   _____

_____   _____

_____   _____

_____   _____

_____   _____

_____   _____

Organizational Chart

Consider a visual that depicts the whole, such as an organizational chart. This is a traditional organizational chart format.

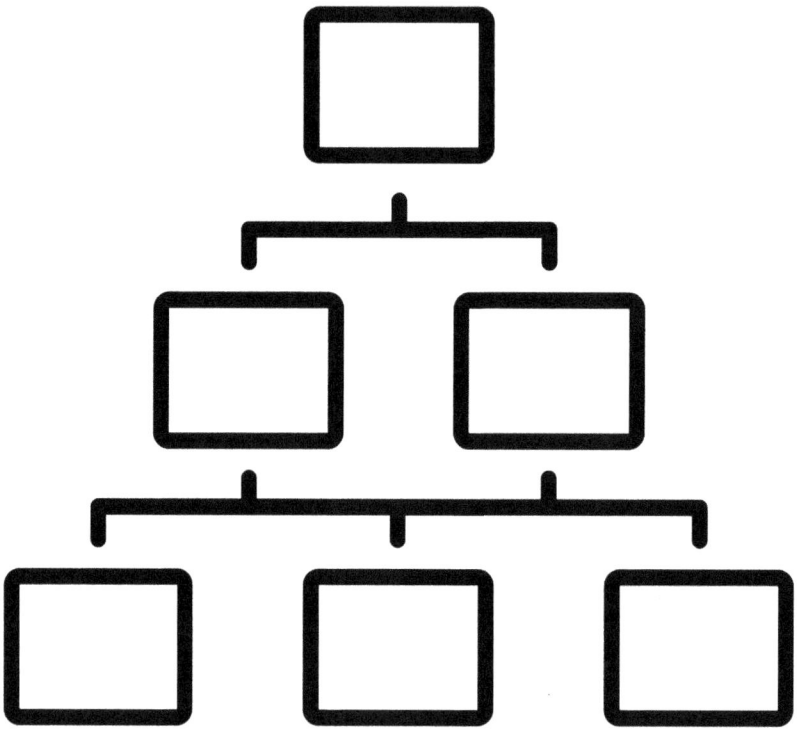

I am not entirely convinced that this traditional organizational chart is accurate for most family caregiving situations. You may be the CEO, but are there really departments and functions, each headed up by a leader or manager? Not typically. (To be honest, I am not sure it suits many businesses and organizations either.)

I have created an organizational chart diagram that I feel might be a bit more accurate for the family caregiving situation. I call it the fan, not for any clever mnemonic or acronym but because of its shape. Who knows? Perhaps the name and shape will also help you keep your cool in difficult situations.

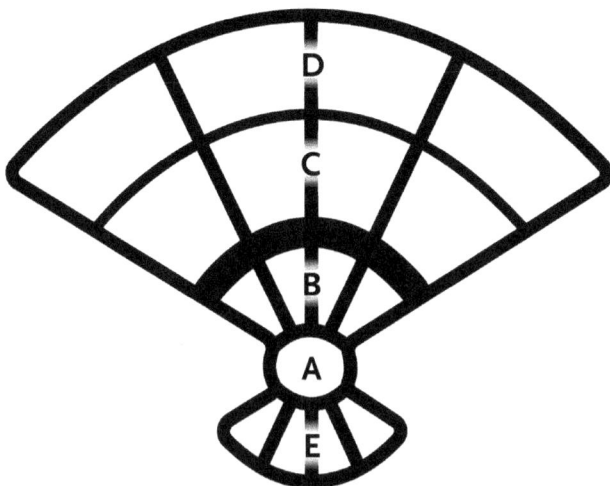

The legend for this format might go something like

A – Your name and the care recipient's name both in the circle at the base.

B – The others who are most dependable in the next tier up, perhaps organized in the sections according to what specifically they are best at or most able to contribute (money/supplies, time, guidance, tasks).

C – In the next tier up, those who occasionally help and must be communicated with. That is, they are stakeholders of sorts, but they may not be as active participants as the first tier.

D – In the very top tier, those who need to be communicated with for periodic updates but really cannot be asked to participate in the care.

E – In the sections below the circle, professional caregivers, such as physicians, social workers, nurses, etc.

Think about how you will inspire and see the people in each part of the fan as individuals. How will you facilitate their caregiving, and how will they interact with you—and perhaps with each other? Have you shared the mission and vision with them? Remember the elements of leadership: Set the vision, bring everything together, and communicate effectively.

Family Caregiver Position Description

> "That's above my pay grade."

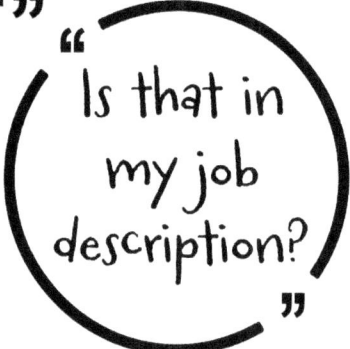

> "Is that in my job description?"

An accurate, comprehensive position description is one of the most essential tools in hiring and management. As a manager, leader, and consultant, I have promoted, recruited, and hired for many positions. I started to think about having to hire for the position of family caregiver. What would that position description look like? I created the position description that follows. You may find this family caregiver position description helpful for a few reasons:

- Validates the magnitude of the family caregiver job.
- Provides professional language and descriptions for the tasks and responsibilities you've become proficient in. This may help if/when you need to describe the position on a résumé or to a future potential employer.
- By considering all the tasks and responsibilities, you may identify opportunities for outsourcing and delegating.

Position descriptions in general are useful tools for leaders. If you find yourself hiring an aide or other professional, consider asking the individual or agency for a position description so that you have a full understanding of the tasks and responsibilities you can expect from the individual. For example, does the aide position include light chores when the care recipient is sleeping or otherwise occupied? Or are you going to be paying an aide to play games on their phone when your care recipient does not have immediate or active help needs?

Position Description

Position title: Family/Uncompensated Caregiver

Responsible to: family, care recipients, physicians, other health care professionals, self, and future self

Position summary: Provide 24/7 in-person or on-call all-round support to loved one, including personal and hygiene needs, health care, food preparation, mobility assistance, emotional support, personal supervision, transportation, recordkeeping, household organization and management, coordination of appointments and external commitments, communication of updates and developments, crisis management, mediation, and end-of-life planning and preparation. May include financial management and/or support.

Educational, license, and certification requirements and preferences: A position description, especially in health care, includes the required and preferred education, licensures, and certifications, typically up toward the top of the document, because if a candidate does not have the necessary education, license, and/or certification, there is no point in pursuing the position. In the case of a family caregiver, some may coincidentally have licenses or certifications, but most do not.

Qualifications and experience: Same as above. A position description would typically include minimum qualifications and experience, such as "three to five years in a management position" or "proven experience _____." While some family caregivers may come into this role with qualifications and experience, most have none, and none are required.

Responsibilities and tasks include but are not limited to:

- Maintains a safe, clean environment at all times (this may include provisions for care recipient with memory or mental cognition deficiencies).

- Administers IM injections, manages wound care, changes dressings, conducts prosthetic care, manages use and maintenance of catheter/port/nutrition devices, cleans and changes urine and colostomy bags.
- Accurately takes (and records as necessary) vital signs, including pulse, temperature, blood pressure, etc.
- Cleans up biohazard materials, including vomit, blood, urine, stool.
- Administers medications in strict accordance with protocols and orders.
- Purchases and manages medical supplies and protects all medications from diversion.
- Prepares meals providing specific dietary needs associated with care recipient's condition/treatment and, if necessary, feeds care recipient.
- (Daily) bathes and (as needed) changes undergarments of care recipient.
- Monitors care recipient for signs of side effects, infection, adverse reactions, discomfort, nutritional needs, and sleep disturbance.
- Schedules and coordinates transportation for all health care and other appointments.
- Maintains health care records, including patient history, adverse reactions, allergies, payer details, medication formularies, and other essential information.
- Participates as needed in insurance prior authorization process as advocate for timely approval.
- Establishes and works within an annual budget.
- Purchases all personal supplies and provisions.
- Manages all accounts payable, financial statements, taxes, health care bills, explanations of benefits (EOBs), etc.
- Records and communicates regular updates as well as alerts/debriefs as to adverse effects and sentinel events with family and other key stakeholders.
- Provides emotional support, including active listening, demonstrated compassion, and sound guidance.

- Stays current on all treatments, clinical trials, recalls, changes in law, resources, and other dynamic aspects of the disease-/condition-specific situation.
- Advocates on behalf of care recipient with physicians, health care professionals, insurance companies and payers, social services, state and local government, and other organizations and individuals as necessary.
- Attends all meetings and health care appointments.
- Attends all training and development made available or required (e.g., hospital discharge).
- Performs additional duties as requested or required by the situation or need.
- Serves as health care proxy, determining, managing, and advocating for care recipient's end-of-life, remains disposition, memorial, and legacy wishes.

Typical physical demands: Position requires full range of body motion, including handling and lifting patient, manual and finger dexterity, and eye-hand coordination. Involves standing and walking. Caregiver will occasionally be asked to lift and carry items weighing up to sixty pounds. Normal visual acuity and hearing are required. Caregiver will work under stressful conditions and work irregular hours. Caregiver will be exposed to bodily fluids on a regular basis. Caregiver will be required to transport patient and must have a valid driver's license and working, properly outfitted vehicle.

Standard working conditions: Caregiver will be present or "on call" 24/7/365 with no breaks unless coverage is secured. Caregiver must work in all locations and conditions, including home, car/public transportation, hospital, clinic, and all other facilities. Frequent exposure to communicable diseases, toxic substances, ionizing radiation, medicinal preparation, and other conditions common to a clinical environment.

Salary/compensation range: Uncompensated.

Professional Caregivers & Palliative Care

Likely, your care recipient sees multiple professional caregivers, such as physicians of various specialties, advanced practice nurses (APNs), physician associate (PAs), nurse practitioners (NPs), nurses, occupational therapists, physical therapists, etc. Include professional caregivers on your list of those who do help.

In my experience, the medical specialty that best recognizes the role of family caregivers is palliative care, which is available in most, although not all, locations. In medicine, the specialty is often called hospice and palliative care, but that does not mean that hospice and palliative care are the same. The two terms are not interchangeable.

All hospice is palliative care.
Not all palliative care is hospice.

- To palliate means to comfort or to make a condition less harsh, harmful, or painful. Care that is palliative eases and alleviates suffering.
- The indication for hospice care is a life expectancy of six months or less. Hospice care is most often provided in the patient's or family's place of residence. Hospice care provides comfort to the patient and support to the family until death. (Hospice also includes thirteen months of bereavement support for the family following the death of the patient.)

Thus, *everything* within hospice is meant to be palliative, to ease suffering, and to lessen pain and symptoms.

However, when someone and their family are *living* with a serious condition, they may need or benefit from the lessening of pain and symptoms even if they are not near end of life. That's palliative care.

Because these two areas of focus in medicine are similar but not the same, and because all of hospice care is palliative in nature, even most health care professionals—including physicians and nurses—

do not truly know the difference and often *incorrectly* treat the two terms, "palliative care" and "hospice," as synonymous and meaning end-of-life care only.

A palliative care (PC) team includes a physician; an advanced practice nurse, nurse practitioner, or physician assistant; a social worker; a chaplain; and often a clinical pharmacist—all subspecialty-trained in PC.

If your care recipient has cancer, ALS, or another life-limiting condition involving multiple specialists and a slew of medications, please ask for a consultation with the PC team. I always say, "Palliative care: Go early, go often." If your care recipient has a life-limiting condition, do not let anyone tell you "It is too soon for PC." When someone tells you "It's too soon for PC" or "We're not there yet," it is an indication that they do not fully understand the difference between PC and hospice as described above. If you are established with PC, go as often as you feel necessary. The website GetPalliativeCare.org will help you find palliative care in your area.

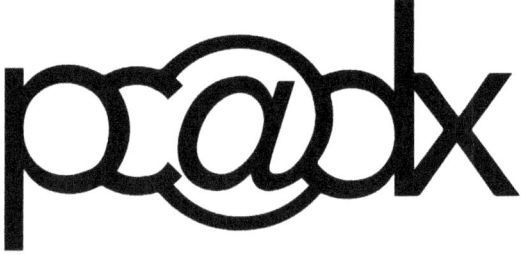

I created the design above, "Palliative Care at Diagnosis," as a reminder that with serious, life-limiting conditions, it is never too early for extra help from the subspecialty known as palliative care.

Advisors

Effective CEOs engage advisors and experts to provide guidance and outsource functions. Here are some advisors you might want to consult.

Patient Advocate: Helps with navigating the health care system. Let's face it: The health care system is vast and complicated, and aspects of it are crucial to carrying out your mission. A patient advocate can help locate necessary services and equipment. They can provide support when you are communicating with third-party payers such as Medicare or an insurance company. There are several ways to locate a patient advocate: You can start with a local hospital, medical center, or physician organization. If that doesn't feel quite right to you, try the Patient Advocate Foundation (PatientAdvocate.org) and the National Patient Advocate Foundation (npaf.org). You can also search online for "patient advocate," along with your location, to see what comes up; many communities have several resources.

Financial Advisor: Provides expert advice on managing personal finances; this may include budgeting, planning, investments, insurance, retirement, and other guidance. Do not think you do not have enough in assets to warrant a good financial advisor; with the costs of health care and the effects of illness on household income, you are at risk for losing what you do have.

Find a financial advisor who will take a holistic approach to your situation and has experience with family caregiving, chronic illness, and life-limiting conditions, as well as estate and end-of-life planning. You might ask if they have clients who are or were in a similar situation who would talk with you as references.

Elder Law Attorney: Handles legal matters affecting an older or disabled person, including issues related to health care, long-term care planning, guardianship, retirement, social security, Medicare, etc. If appropriate, get an elder law attorney with expertise in veterans' affairs benefits and appeals.

Geriatric Care Manager: Advocates for and guides those caring for older and/or disabled adults. They are educated and experienced in several fields, including counseling, gerontology, mental health, nursing, educational therapy, physical therapy, psychology, and social work. They have a specialized focus on issues related to aging and elder care. You may hire this type of advisor on an hourly basis. The Aging Life Care Association (AgingLifeCare.org) offers guidance and referrals related to these professionals.

Doula: This term means "companion" or "helper." You may be familiar with obstetrics doulas, people who are experienced and trained to provide advice, information, and support during pregnancy and birth. There is a growing field of end-of-life doulas. An end-of-life doula in your local area can be an outstanding resource, especially as your care recipient gets closer to death. I am not sure it is ever too early to start considering which end-of-life doula might be available and a good fit for your situation. Beyond a general web search, several national and international organizations can help locate end-of-life doulas, including:

- International End-of-Life Doula Association (inelda.org)
- National End-of-Life Doula Association (NEDAlliance.org)
- Doulagivers Institute (Doulagivers.com)

As you select and work with any of these types of advisors, some general advice applies:

- Be selective when considering different advisors. Whenever possible, shop and compare services and pricing.
- While you may be asked to sign a release to hold them harmless or to acknowledge a description of their services, there should be no need to sign a contract with any of these types of advisors.
- Insist that your advisor explain what they're doing and why—whenever necessary, and as often as necessary.
- Make sure you feel comfortable with them. If you don't feel comfortable at any point, let them know, and, if necessary, discontinue the service.

Family/Circle

The family—that dear octopus from whose tentacles we never quite escape, nor, in our inmost hearts, ever quite wish to.

—Dodie Smith

A sibling who doesn't help with the caregiving of a parent when and how you need them to is no less a son or a daughter of the care recipient. It's a frustration akin to a board member who doesn't show up to the meetings, or who plays on their mobile device throughout a long, involved discussion and then wants everything to stop just before the important vote because they need more information about the issue.

One difference is that family members don't rotate off as board members may.

These are challenging aspects of the caregiver-as-leader position when you must facilitate, inspire, finesse, and perhaps even manipulate (a little) to get the participation you need, or at least to minimize the disruption or paralysis resulting from a lack of participation.

Here again, if you have already established the mission, vision, and values, share them and get some input on what other family members might add. If you have not yet established the mission, vision, and values, consider inviting all family members to participate in the conversation. If some family members are long-distance, send emails asking for words and phrases that should be included, and give them a date when you are going to start to put it all together so that they have a timeline. Send first drafts of the mission and vision statements and get input and suggestions. Tweak and send subsequent draft(s) until you feel you have final mission and vision statements, and then share those.

However you go about establishing the mission, vision, values, and (perhaps) mantra, as a CEO you will need to share them repeatedly.

Keeping these ideals in view is part of leadership, and it helps people feel they're a part of something larger than themselves. Remember: Lead in a way that inspires people to realize that the whole is indeed greater than the sum of its parts.

Meetings & Communication

Accept that family/circle members are going to talk among themselves, just like employees have conversations that leave out management. It's okay; in fact, it can be extremely fruitful.

Hold or offer regular meetings—perhaps once monthly or quarterly—in person or by video conferencing. And while you certainly don't need to follow *Robert's Rules of Order*, a family meeting is different from a catch-up call. It's more like a business meeting.

Business meetings typically have:

- A set time, location, and duration.
- A realistic agenda. The first five sections of this book (Strategy & Planning; Team & Resources; Data & Analysis; Facility, Environmental Services & Supplies; and Self-Management) might work as a standing agenda outline and a framework for participants' additions of agenda items before the meeting.
- A facilitative leader. This person leads the group through the agenda and facilitates the conversation and contributions. The CEO is not always the meeting leader. Sometimes a meeting is more productive and effective if someone else leads.
- A timekeeper. This individual keeps an eye on the clock, with the goal of getting the entire agenda covered during the allotted time. For example, if the meeting were scheduled for one hour and there were six equally important/dense items on the agenda, the timekeeper would try to keep the discussions to ten minutes each. If one topic were weightier or more urgent, they might cover that item at the beginning and

allocate fifteen minutes, taking five minutes from something that is likely to be quicker.
- A recordkeeper who keeps some notes on decisions and tracks follow-up.
- A follow-up communication that highlights the discussions, decisions, assignments, and other specifics. (This might be akin to meeting minutes and can be used at a subsequent meeting as a starting point.)

If your circle/family is not used to this type of meeting and the first one doesn't run on time or gets sidetracked, don't give up. These types of implementations take time and effort to make work. As the caregiving needs and situation intensify, you will likely benefit from having established and honed the meeting process.

Sample Family/Circle Meeting Agenda

Regular Family Meeting Regarding Care for _____

Date: Duration:

Time: Place:

- Welcome—Review Mission and Vision (2 minutes)
- Strategy & Planning (0 minutes)
- Team & Resources (5 minutes)
    - Introduce SupportNow.org and how it can be used for everyone to participate.
    - Finalize plans for coverage during the upcoming trip—primary family caregiver has to take kid to college.
- Data & Analysis (15 minutes)
    - Significant changes to routines or methods and the results (e.g., the days are getting shorter, so sundown syndrome is affecting our care recipient's behavior earlier and earlier each day; we've made an adjustment to medication timing or dose; etc.).
    - Upcoming expenses or budget issues.
- Facility, Environmental Services & Supplies (15 minutes)

- The doctor suggested a walker might help with ambulation.
- Feeling the need to increase the number of times the cleaning service comes.
- Repairs that are needed to domicile and plans to get them done with minimal disruption.
- Self-Management (5 minutes)
    - Thanks to _____ for covering last Friday afternoon so I could have an afternoon to myself. We may need to start doing something like this once a _____. Can we develop a schedule for that?
- Other Business (5 minutes)
- If possible, gather Other Business items ahead of time and list them here.
- The next meeting is at (time), on (day of week), (date).
- Adjourn

This is a sample agenda for a regular meeting. By meeting periodically, you are involving others all along the way so that when major changes or decisions need to be made, the group is accustomed to meeting, discussing, and deciding.

Listening

Listening is essential to effective leadership. More minds are better than one, people need to be heard to feel a part of something, and they may in fact have valuable contributions to make. As caregivers and leaders, it is to our advantage to listen politely, sort through the parlance, and parse out good ideas from quiet discards.

On average, adults conversationally speak 120 to 150 words per minute.[6] Our thoughts, however, have an average rate of several hundred (up to 800) words per minute.[7] Recognizing and managing the vast gap between the number of words a person can say to you and the number of words you are naturally capable of processing while they are speaking is an essential component to effective listening. We must slow our brains down from those several hundred words that naturally zoom through our minds per minute and focus on the mere 135 that are being spoken—each and every minute of the conversation.

Think about the implications that this gap has on your ability to listen and take in information. When a physician tells of a new diagnosis or comorbidities, this gap may increase with fast, anxious thoughts of uncertainty, dread, and/or overwhelm. When a non-contributing family member decides it is time to call you and offer thoughts or suggestions, this gap may be filled with resentment, anger, and/or distraction.

Yet, listening is an essential element of effective leadership and family caregiving. Knowing about this gap will help you slow your mind down to focus on the words, meanings, intonations, facts, and messages being spoken. Here are some tactics that might help:

Determine if the conversation can be scheduled or managed via written communication.

---

[6] Dom Barnard, "Average Speaking Rate and Words per Minute," *Virtual Speech* (November 2022).
[7] Speakeasy, "Are You Really Listening: Listening vs. Hearing" (June 2004).

Listen to understand rather than to respond or rebut. This one is especially important in troubled relationships or during tension or conflict.

Have a pen and paper or device handy so that you can make notes, which will slow your thoughts down.

Don't feel as though you must respond immediately; take time to process what is being said. Acknowledge that you have heard and need some time to process and think.

Utilize the teach-back method to ensure and demonstrate that you have heard and understood accurately and completely. Listen until the end, then ask permission to restate what you believe you've just learned to ensure thorough and accurate understanding.

- For example: Thanks for calling. This sounds like an interesting idea. Let me repeat back to you what I've heard and think you are suggesting so we can both be sure I understand.

Friends & Stakeholders

Occasionally, as CEO, I get help from some indirect or unlikely sources—perhaps a vendor or a community leader whose organization or business has a stake or general interest in my organization doing well.

Sometimes just letting a friend know of a challenging situation yields help. This is one place where people's overwhelming desire to "fix it" can be parlayed into delegation and other assistance.

Don't forget your care recipient's friends. When I was family caregiver to my mother as she died of cancer, in addition to her siblings, several of her close friends came forward one after another to help. Some of her friends helped me communicate with other friends whom I did not know how to contact. Sometimes my mother's friends sat with her when I needed a break.

As my mother neared death, I was certain that she didn't want to be alone, but also that she didn't want me to be the one at her side. She had protected me from that sort of intense, difficult experience for most of my life, and she was not going to make an exception for her own death. As the active dying process began, she went into that deep sleep with the very loud breathing (not snoring), frequently referred to as the death rattle, which is common in the active dying process. I wondered and worried about how someone who loved her would be there with her if it wasn't going to be me. The more I tried to stay with her, the more certain I was that she didn't want me there, so I left. Sure enough, one of her oldest and dearest friends arrived from across the country just hours before she took her last breath and was, quite simply, the perfect person to be there with her as she died.

Think about friends (yours and your care recipient's), their strengths and interests, and how they might fit an additional need.

Delegation

"Let me know if there is anything I can do to help."

No doubt the phrase above is one you have heard and will continue to hear, especially after you communicate updates and developments. Hearing this as a caregiver can feel frustrating, perhaps useless. So often, this offer makes the speaker feel better (they have offered help!) and puts the burden on the receiver of the offer. It is the *receiver* who must identify needs and then express them.

Yet, when leaders hear, "Let me know if there is anything I can do to help," they follow up with an answer. So when friends, relations, and acquaintances say, "Let me know if there is anything I can do," let them know. You are, after all, the CEO. While some people say that reflexively with no real notion of helping, many people mean it, which makes it an opportunity for you to delegate a task or responsibility.

Effective delegation is a key aspect of leadership. When someone says, "Let me know what I can do to help," and you know they mean it, you do not have to have an answer on the spot. Think about an appropriate task for them, and then follow up. Text something like this:

Wonderful to run into you the other day. Thanks for your offer to help.

If you are still up for it, I have an idea of something that would make a huge difference for us and will hopefully be easy for you. If not, I understand. Let me know.

Websites such as SupportNow.org,* LotsaHelpingHands.com, and CircleOf.com allow friends, family, and others to participate in organized support such as meals, visits, and rides to medical appointments. When someone says, "Let me know what I can do to help," text them a link to your page on one of the support websites so they can sign on, participate, and commit to what best suits them.

---

* SupportNow.org is the preferred support coordination system because it is free and makes communication, meal provision, task coordination, and fundraising available in one place, which is more efficient for both the host of the page and the supporters.

People who have been through something like what you are going through are often the best helpers. So just because someone is a mere acquaintance, do not write them off as a possible support source and delegation opportunity.

Reluctant to delegate? First, let's start with the most common reasons people do not delegate:

- Believing it takes less time to just do the task oneself than it does to explain.
- Feeling guilty about asking someone else to do a job or take over a responsibility.
- Thinking the other person won't do as good a job with it.
- Being overly specific about method and just how the task needs to be done.

Does any of this sound familiar? It does to me; I have certainly used one or more of these excuses on occasion.

Frequently, family caregivers feel that if they delegate, they are shirking responsibility or losing control. To be an effective leader, it is essential to get your altitude up and see the bigger picture so you don't burn out or make yourself ill. As we explored earlier in this section, there *are* people who can, will, and want to help. This is true even when it feels to the family caregiver that no one else can help.

Leaders do not do every job in the organizations they lead. Leadership demands delegation, collaboration, and communication. I have known a couple of CEOs who kept critical tasks to themselves, and they remained CEOs for only a short time.

Family caregivers do a lot. They may even do most of the work. But family caregivers cannot possibly do it all. You simply will not fully realize the mission and vision and enjoy some of the Precious Time if you alone are consumed by every single one of the tasks and responsibilities.

Initiating Delegation

Initially, effective delegation takes time and effort. It gets easier with this three-step process:

- Determine which tasks and responsibilities can be delegated.
- Identify who is best to take over the task or responsibility.
- Communicate what is needed and any timing or deadline issues clearly.

Let's go through each of the three steps in detail.

1. Determine Tasks & Responsibilities to Delegate

Write each task you are considering delegating on a sticky note or an index card. If you need help making a list of tasks and responsibilities, reference the caregiver position description earlier in this section. Next, on a wallboard, desk, table, or door, create three sections with headings: "Retain" for those tasks you will keep; "Delegate" for those responsibilities you will give entirely to someone else; and "Share" for anything you are considering completing with someone else.

Take some time with this process. Be bold and move the tasks back and forth among the three columns to determine where each best belongs.

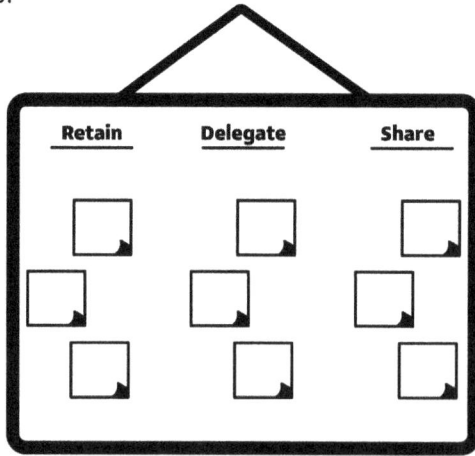

2. Identify Who Is Best for Each Task

Whether you go by personality assessment tool or astrological sign or you just know your peeps, as a leader you learn that different individuals are suited to and comfortable with different types of tasks and efforts. Try thinking of the people in your circle in terms of the following categories. Which type of motivation is most important to each of them?

- **Social (S):** The person who is always planning the next potluck or birthday celebration and does so because they enjoy relationships, networking, and socializing.
- **Driven (D):** The one who wants to know if it has ever been done before, or ever been done this fast or effectively, and who has a drive toward accomplishment—perhaps even some sense of competition.
- **Independent (I):** The individual who just wants to know what you want done and by when and then wants to be left alone to do it. They don't like to be managed, much less micromanaged.
- **Steady On (SO):** The folks who do not like change and uncertainty; they prioritize creating an atmosphere of comfort, security, and consistency.
- **Persuasive (P):** Those who are driven by the ability to persuade and convince others.

The simplified motivation style summary above combines several assessment instruments and leadership education I have been fortunate enough to be exposed to. It includes impressions from the DISC assessment, Development Dimensions International, the Myers Briggs Type Indicator, as well as decades of my own leadership experience.

Next, think about what each person is proficient in and enjoys. Make a list of people in your circle, and note each person's motivation type and/or proficiencies on the next page:

Name	Motivation Type (S, D, I, SO, or P) and/or Proficiency

Once you have taken care to list tasks to delegate and identify people you will delegate to, begin to design your delegation by writing a name on each sticky note or index card. Match each task to a person with capabilities that fit well, and highlight aspects of the responsibility that speak to their qualities.

For example, perhaps one friend is independently motivated, is great at evaluating information, and spends a lot of time on YouTube. You need training tools for giving intramuscular injections for a new medication your care recipient may soon require. Ask that person to research training videos and identify the top two or three for you to review.

3. Communicate Clearly, Including Deadlines

In the next section, Data & Analysis, we'll cover the urgent/important matrix. Use that as your guide when establishing and communicating deadlines and check-in points for individual tasks and projects. Especially if something is important but not urgent, a single deadline may not provide enough information, so suggest dates or points in the process for progress check-ins.

Communicate the differences between hard deadlines and soft ones. A soft deadline might be a time/date when you would really *like* something to be complete, while a hard deadline is the date by which it *must* be complete.

Communicate and check in periodically. Recognize that those who have a preference for independence will respond less well to frequent check-ins, so assign them tasks and projects that require less of that. Having said that, no one likes to feel micromanaged, so if a need to control and direct is an issue for you, let go of some of that.

Overcoming Conflict & Obstacles

In addition to leading a group, a CEO leads each individual and may need to get involved in relationships between two or three individuals within the group or team.

Ideas for overcoming conflict and obstacles:

- Recognize that the overall mission and vision and several inherent aspects of caregiving (including end of life, finances, medications, and past relationships) are highly emotionally charged for everyone involved.
- Determine whether there are any communication gaps: "Did you receive the last email update? Let me send it so we all have the same information."
- Approach each person with curiosity rather than judgment (even if you have known the person all their life and think you know enough to judge).
- Find common ground and opportunities.
- Ask what their biggest concerns are, and then listen without interruption to the answers.
- Ask for their ideas for solutions, and then listen without interruption to the answers.
- Revisit the mission, vision, and core values.
- Ask, "What is your mantra for this situation?" Listen and consider their response. Then, perhaps, add yours. This communication starter may help illuminate where there are differences and opportunities.
- Give them a copy of this book so they understand the leadership perspective and some of the tools you are using.
- Apologize when it is warranted. (Overusing "I'm sorry" can dilute its meaning; if you save it for the times when you truly need or want to apologize, it will remain more powerful and genuine.)
- Listen and acknowledge apologies when they are offered. Indicate your acceptance or lack of acceptance of an apology.

Pinpointed Positive Feedback & Thank Yous

Detailed, positive feedback is one of the best tools in a leader's toolbox—I kid you not. But it must be specific. "Good job" or "Way to go!" is nice to hear, but it does not tell the individual what was effective about the action taken.

After that visit from the sister who rarely finds time to come and sit with Mom so you can have an afternoon off, send her a text that says, "Thanks so much for taking care of Mom this afternoon. You must have gotten some quality time with her, because she was particularly calm and content later in the day. It was so nice of you to straighten up the place and empty the dishwasher. It gave me some extra time to sort out the medications when I got home."

Positive feedback and expressed gratitude typically beget more of the same behavior. And remember that positives can be shared openly. When others overhear your praise, the specifics will help them understand what exactly is helpful. When helpers receive positive feedback from you, they will be more open to conversing about how they can improve or be of still greater assistance.

As you give clear, specific, positive feedback, perhaps tie it into support of the mission, vision, or values when appropriate. People love to be part of something larger than themselves, and effective leaders help them know they are at every possible opportunity.

A note here on another use for "thank you." Lately, I have been converting what starts in my head as "Sorry for _____ (the delay, tardiness, confusion, mixed signals)" to "Thank you for your patience," and I think it is infinitely more effective in a few ways. It doesn't set me up as inadequate or substandard from the start. The word "patience" places value on what is really needed and appreciated. Credit for the patience is well placed and involves the other person as an active participant rather than a passive recipient. It's a positive reframe. And finally, it doesn't dilute the impact of a true apology. "I'm sorry," as I've mentioned, has become a filler phrase in our conversational language. When we clutter our conversations with trite uses of "I'm sorry," true apologies lose some of their power and importance. "Thank you for your patience" rather than "I'm sorry" seems an effective conversion of phrasing for both caregivers and leaders.

Communication

Some of the most important lessons I learned in my early days of leadership were related to effective communication with key stakeholders. Here are some of the specifics:

- Get ahead of questions and doubts while staying in the front of people's minds by communicating clearly even when the update is that there's nothing new to report.
- Keep communication concise. Long emails do not get read in their entirety. Begin with something friendly and thoughtful and then **get to the point**.
- Put the most important stuff early in the written communication.
- Communicate in the modality most likely to be received. Some older folks need you to use your phone *as a phone*. If they *must* get the information, use their preferred communication method.
- Don't lie or fudge the truth; it is disrespectful and destroys your credibility.
- If one person asks a question or demonstrates a lack of understanding, it indicates that others may have similar questions and thus may be a reason for an update or clarification.
- Be inclusive.
- Written communication does not come with facial expression, voice tone, inflection, or gestures. The reader will likely default to the negative—that's just human nature. Sarcasm and opacity have no place in any type of written communication.
- Don't address one or two individuals' counterproductive or negative behavior with a group email; speak to them directly and privately. If you make a "general announcement" about something that only one or two people are doing, those who are doing it will not realize it is directed at them, and those who are not engaged in the behavior will become confused or unappreciative of the direction.
- Sometimes long distribution lists get ignored by many of

the recipients. Recipients see that many others are getting the message, and they may feel that since someone else will pay attention, they themselves don't really need to. I have been known to cut and paste super important stuff and send out individual emails or texts with added personalization to ensure the recipients each sense they are depended upon.

Resources

We are so fortunate to have automation, websites, and apps available to facilitate our caregiving mission and vision. The following are just a few resources available to family caregivers:

Illness-specific organizations: If your care recipient has a specific diagnosis such as Alzheimer's, ALS, a particular type of cancer, Parkinson's disease, etc., please check out the illness-specific organizations that apply and access their resources and support groups.

AngelSense: A GPS tracker for those with dementia and other special needs.

Caregiving.com: A community for family caregivers.

TheConversationProject.org: A trove of conversation starters and guides for end-of-life preparation, including guides for special circumstances, such as a care recipient with dementia.

Insurance or government payer apps: If your care recipient has health insurance through a company or Medicare replacement plan, please check out which apps and resources that company makes available to their members. There are typically resources included.

YourELDR.com: This network of professionals will connect you with an elder to take you from zero to completely end of life—ready in eight virtual visits. They have elders who specialize in all cultures and needs and are adept at working with individuals and families after serious illness has been diagnosed and become a factor in end-of-life preparation and planning.

SupportNow.org: Provides and coordinates the four major areas of support that family caring situations need. It's a communication tool that allows one to update others in the wider circle (similar to CaringBridge.org); a task assignment system like LotsaHelpingHands.com; a meal scheduling and provision system akin to Meal-

Train.com; and a fundraising site similar to (but with fewer charges than) GoFundMe.com.

Wellthy.com: A care coordination service that helps families organize and support their caregiving. You can enter questions or lists of what you need help with, and their professionals will respond. An example: "I need help finding an oncologist for my mom, sorting through a bill from a recent hospital stay, ordering prescriptions, and someone to help her at home in the evenings."

Because of the dynamic nature of technology and web-based resources, please check out JenniferAOBrien.com/Resources for more information.

Social Media

Wise leaders find their people for support, information, connection, and humor. Individuals and organizations on various social media platforms offer guidance and connection for family caregivers. Many of these offer content that covers more than one category.

Because social media accounts are dynamic, please visit JenniferAOBrien.com/Resources for an up-to-date list of family caregiver resources in the following categories:

- Family caregiving (general)
- Dementia care
- Hospice and end of life
- Palliative care
- End-of-life planning
- Chronic conditions

Search on your preferred social media platforms for specific illnesses, conditions, locations, and questions to find appropriate resources. My preferred social media platforms are Instagram, Facebook, and LinkedIn, so many of the accounts I have made available to you on the resources page of my website can be found on those. Many organizations and individuals provide the same or similar information on all mainstream social media platforms.

3

Data & Analysis

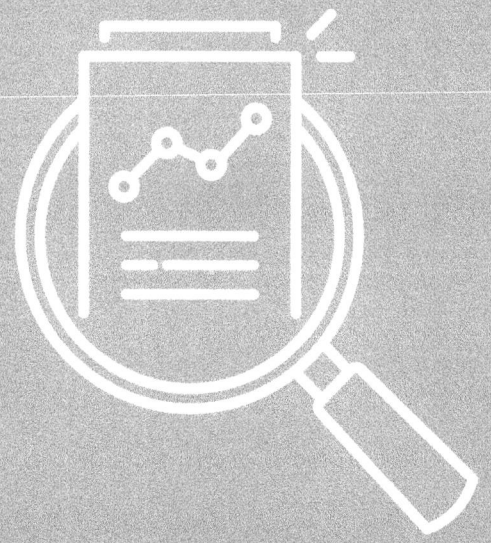

New Message

To: Family Caregiver

Subject: Using my brain to analyze data helps my heart

Dear Caregiver,

Within Bob's and my marriage, I was the one who paid the bills, managed maintenance, hired contractors when we needed them, etc. I ran the household, planned the trips, and did the overall administrative work. He was as involved as I needed him to be, but mostly these sorts of decisions and management were up to me.

When he became ill, however, he kept strict control of the medications. He was, after all, a physician, and the responsibility for and proper handling of medications and controlled substances had been second nature to him for nearly five decades. Of course, I deferred to him, even though there were times when he would try to wean himself off a pain medication and end up suffering (i.e., super crabby), and I would realize something was going on and ask him how it was going with his pain, to which he would sheepishly confess that he had been scaling back and was suffering because of it.

Shortly after he was admitted to hospice status in our home, the nurse kindly and privately told me that with the additional medications from hospice and his decline, she felt he was no longer able to manage them himself. I guess I knew this was coming, yet it was terribly upsetting to me. Here was the one thing that was totally second nature to him for years and years, and as he got sicker, he was unable to do it himself.

That night after Bob fell asleep, I cried and cried at the fact that my husband, who had taken great care and pride in his commitment to being a physician, was slipping away and no longer able to manage one of the most basic tasks of that profession.

After a good cry, I realized that the medication management was a matter of data, dosing, and schedule. I spread all the drugs and related supplies out on the kitchen table, got out my phone and a pad of paper, and started to look up each and every drug brand name and generic name, purpose, and dose. This was data. I could study it and learn it, and then I would know how to administer the medications safely and effectively. It felt good to use my brain, to process information objectively. There is no subjectivity or feeling in the fact that ondansetron/Zofran is taken to help with nausea and vomiting; that is a fact. It was refreshing to be working in data, information, analysis, and scheduling. It was head work rather than heart work. There is no subjectivity in a baseline pain medication schedule and if you miss giving the medication, the pain will get worse. So, I made a schedule, set timers on my phone (time—completely objective) and managed the medications schedule. Ironically, it *felt* good to be using my brain rather than my heart.

I have always said that success calls for a balance of head and heart every day. We put a lot of heart into caregiving, but to really lead we need some head too.

As I said, I see you. I also understand you, support you, and love you.

—jennifer

It is a capital mistake to theorize before one has data.

—Arthur Conan Doyle, *Sherlock Holmes*

There are only two ways to enhance the bottom line:

- Reduce expen$e$
- Increa$e revenue$

When it comes to money there is no subjectivity. There are funds in and funds out. The only way to improve the net situation is to bring in more and/or to spend less.

That's it. Only two ways. One of the reasons I love coming back to financials and other data is their objectivity. There is absolutely nothing subjective about the bottom line. This is as true for CEOs of Fortune 500 companies as it is for family caregivers. It is another universal truth.

The contents of this section:

- Budgeting
- Reporting Periods
- Data-Based Decisions
- Goals
- Treatment Decisions
- Root Cause Analysis
- Urgent/Important Matrix
- The Immeasurable

Budgeting

Every CEO worth their salt begins a fiscal year with a detailed budget projection. There are two parts to a detailed budget projection:

- The budgeted or projected revenue/income.
- The budgeted or projected expenses.

Use a spreadsheet program, such as Microsoft Excel or Numbers, or a budgeting app to get started. Enter the projected income from all the regular sources. Next, based on existing bills, complete the section on what the projected expenses are likely to be.

If you have never done such a budgeting process, keep in mind that it can be daunting, but don't give up on it. Start by simply listing everything, using the amounts you have spent in the past. It's best to start with a typical month and then continue through the year to account for expenses that only come up quarterly or annually.

The income minus the expenses equals the bottom line. The bottom line may be a positive number or a negative number. If it's a negative number, it is considered a deficit. After your initial completion of the budget, if the bottom line is a deficit, then you need to go back up to the various expenses and see where there are opportunities for reduction or elimination, or identify additional income.

Because revenue rarely increases in a family caregiving situation, expenses must be closely examined regularly. Periodically compare actual expenses to the projected expenses you put in your budget. This will help you make decisions more effectively. For example, you might look at the expense of $250 per month for cable television (for a care recipient who doesn't understand or even notice the television anymore) and decide that money is better spent on a few hours with an advisor, or on a hired caregiver visit that allows a weekly afternoon off for the family caregiver.

Sharing the budget projections and actual income and expenses with those in the family/circle means being open to others' thoughts, inquiries, and suggestions. It also means you're presenting them with objective information that may demonstrate the need for additional funds. Some members of the family/circle may be in a position to contribute additional funds and will appreciate the clear, objective information.

Reporting Periods

Another important element of leadership is reporting periods. As each month, quarter, and year ends, the financials and other data for the period are compiled, reviewed, and compared to projections. As discussed earlier, leaders and family caregivers can get marred by the day-to-day or the grind of it all. Periodically they need to access objective data to gain perspective on the realities and well-being of the endeavor.

In the CEO world, monthly, quarterly, and fiscal year reviews are scheduled in advance. Here again, there is comfort in the fact that time is entirely objective. If you can set up a monthly or quarterly review meeting/call with an advisor, do it. These twelve monthly and/or four quarterly reporting-period reviews help family caregivers and CEOs increase their altitude, thereby enhancing their perspective, learning from the past, and looking toward the future.

Unlike in some other businesses or organizations, in family caregiving it likely makes sense to count the fiscal year (FY) as beginning January 1 and ending December 31. Toward the end of each FY, leaders establish projected expense and revenue budgets for the upcoming year and do an annual report for the previous year. You do not need to print a full-color document here, but make a list of the accomplishments and other factors that support both the mission and the vision of the family caregiving endeavor. This is a way to highlight accomplishments as well as help with making and adjusting plans.

The illustration includes an entire January 1 to December 31 FY divided by quarter, month, and day. I find it valuable to be able to see the month, quarter, and year at a glance, especially when I am making plans or need a broader perspective. How long until the next imaging scan to learn about disease progression? When are the next quarterly estimated taxes due? Which personal events (birthdays, anniversaries) are coming up, and when are the best times for visits from out-of-town family members?

	January	February	March
Q1			

	April	May	June
Q2			

	July	August	September
Q3			

	October	November	December
Q4			

Consider scheduling family/circle meetings to occur just after these reporting periods are complete so that the data from a full month, quarter, or year can be reviewed at some or all the meetings.

Data-Based Decisions

When the mission and vision are laden with emotion and subjectivity, as they are in a family caregiving situation, instances that allow for data-based decisions can be a welcome shift to objectivity and standard performance norms.

Noticing the pattern of your care recipient's anxiety rising at a certain time of day—and adjusting the schedule to help alleviate the agitation and soothe—is a data-based decision.

Determining that getting specialty coffee shop drinks only on weekends would free up the funds to purchase a GPS app subscription for the safety of a care recipient with dementia who is still mobile is also a data-based decision.

In caregiving, we can adopt the same practices that make for effective data use in other fields. For example, when making changes to medications, regimens, or routines that directly impact your care recipient's quality of life or comfort, best practice is to make only one change at a time. That way, you can observe the effects and distinguish causation. For example, if the dosing of two different medications is changed at the same time and there is an adverse effect, it is difficult to tell which change was the cause.

Data-based decisions can be comforting, since most of the other stuff family caregivers deal with is so fraught with emotion.

Goals

A leader measures success using performance goals and indicators. Here again, there is some objectivity in this approach—a quality that may benefit a family caregiver.

While it is not wise to defer emotion in favor of empty busyness, the process and sense of completion related to these more objective tasks and goals can be quite therapeutic, in my experience. And you get stuff done in the process.

Here are some projects and performance indicators that tie directly to caregiving:

- Complete the At Peace Tool Kit (in the Strategy & Planning section) or comprehensive end-of-life plan.
- Declutter, purge, organize, and clean (one closet, storage locker, etc.).
- Organize data and information.
- Implement app/website use so that more people can participate in care and communication.
- Onboard reluctant app or tech users who are key to the caregiving effort.
- Establish your chosen financial management software or app and load the data.
- Schedule, prepare for, and lead a family/circle meeting.
- Complete the medical records file and stock the go bag. (See Strategy & Planning section for more information on this.)

Treatment Decisions

Our health care system and culture tend toward "more is better" and "what can we try next?" This is helpful when there is a possibility of a cure and/or effective disease management. All the treatments in the world, however, will not preclude death, and many of them result in side effects that compromise quality of life.

Because Bob was a physician, he was especially adept at evaluating each of the new treatments that the oncologist proposed for his cancer to determine if he wanted to try them. He did this about five times throughout the course of his illness. Each time one medication stopped working or had an adverse effect, a new medication was proposed, and Bob would evaluate it thoroughly. I have distilled his method down to terms understandable by those of us who did not graduate from medical school.

Unless you are in the emergency department or operating room, you should be able to slow things down and take the time to consider a new treatment. You will *need* to facilitate and/or make treatment decisions with deliberation if you are the activated health care proxy. The first step in such a decision-making process is knowing the treatment's overall objective.

What is the purpose of the treatment?

Cure the disease or condition.

Or

Slow disease progression, possibly prolonging the time before death.

Or

Palliate or make the patient more comfortable by alleviating pain or other symptoms.

There have been numerous studies of patients and their family caregivers to determine if they understand the true goal of the treatment they are receiving. These studies have revealed time and time again that patients and families often think the treatments they receive are curative, even when they are palliative. Calling something a treatment does not mean it is curative or even extends life. It may help alleviate a symptom or side effect, or it may provide comfort or alleviate suffering.

Ask, ask again, and make notes. Do what you need to do to fully understand the objective of each treatment. Learn the possible adverse effects and side effects of the treatments, as well as how likely those effects are. This information is readily available; find it, read it, and consider it. Are the potential side effects worth the possibility of more time? For example, Mom has cancer, and everyone wants to see her at your sister's wedding. Given her condition, is the risk of the side effects for that medication worth it for that goal?

Unless there is an adjunct relationship between two medications (meaning they are required to always be given together), it is ill-advised to make more than one change to the medication regimen at the same time. If more than one adjustment is made at a time and there is a side or adverse effect, there will be a question as to *which* medication change has caused it. Of course, physicians know this, but it is a good idea for the family caregiver to keep this guideline in mind.

There is also the issue of "disease fatigue," which means feeling finished or wanting a break from treatments and side effects. Sometimes people decide to forego treatments that might extend their life and opt for simply being as comfortable as they can be before they die. This is *not* giving up; this is a pivot to concentrating efforts on a peaceful, comfortable remainder of life, then death. This is entering Precious Time. Focusing on comfort does not cause or hasten death. Death happens regardless of what we focus on, talk about, or wish for. A desire or decision to focus on only comfort care will involve either palliative care or hospice, depending on the life expectancy of your care recipient.

Root Cause Analysis

When a significant, suboptimal outcome occurs once or repeatedly, leaders are often called upon to determine what went wrong by doing a root cause analysis. One favorite root cause analysis method is called five whys.[8] It's efficient, effective, and, well, simple. Try it by clearly stating what happened, then following up with the question "Why?" for at least five rounds to realize the root cause.

Debriefing and examining the root cause following a significant event (that went either well or disastrously) is an essential part of leadership. The post-incident analysis helps to avoid the same mistakes or build on successes, and learn from the past.

A TRAFFIC VIOLATION FOR ROLLING A STOP SIGN

1. **Why did I roll the stop sign?**
   I was late driving my care recipient to a doctor's appointment.

2. **Why was I late driving my care recipient to a doctor's appointment?**
   I ended up leaving home later than planned.

3. **Why did I end up leaving home later than planned?**
   I had to find the cold weather gear and scrape the windshield, so it took longer to load up the car and pull out of the driveway.

4. **Why did I have to find the cold weather gear?**
   I was surprised by and unprepared for the freezing precipitation.

5. **Why was I surprised by and unprepared for the freezing precipitation?**
   I did not look at the weather prediction and prepare.

A takeaway for the future might be to check the weather and/or other travel hindrances when an appointment reminder appears or when planning for going out.

---

[8] Sakichi Toyoda, the Japanese industrialist, developed the five whys technique in the 1930s, and it is still used worldwide today.

Urgent/Important Matrix

In 1954, President Dwight D. Eisenhower famously said, "I have two types of problems, the urgent and the important." This certainly feels true for the family caregiver as well.

Eisenhower went on to develop a four-quadrant model (shown on the following page) to help determine what is truly important and urgent as each task or situation arises.

Take a look at the diagram. Tasks or situations in the upper left quadrant are both urgent and important and therefore must be done immediately. These tasks or situations are quite rare; your care recipient falls or has difficulty breathing, or another medical emergency occurs. Respond to these important and urgent situations appropriately and immediately.

The upper right quadrant is for stuff that is important but not urgent; a good example would be working on end-of-life documents. You will work on them steadily as you have time and complete them. The lower left quadrant is for less important tasks with some urgency. Maybe your favorite treat is on sale at the local shop for a limited time. It feels pressing, but it will not yield disaster if you miss it. Delegate this to your bestie and ask them to run by and pick some up for you on sale.

The lower right quadrant is for things that seem important and/or urgent but are neither. They could be hyped-up, in-the-moment tasks, perhaps because of someone's mistake, poor planning, procrastination, lack of communication, stubbornness, or other counterproductive tendencies or behaviors. Identify these core issues as neither urgent nor important, then manage or eliminate them.

This urgent/important matrix is an effective tool for assessing the true nature of a task, situation, or problem—as it arises or as part of a debrief after the fact.

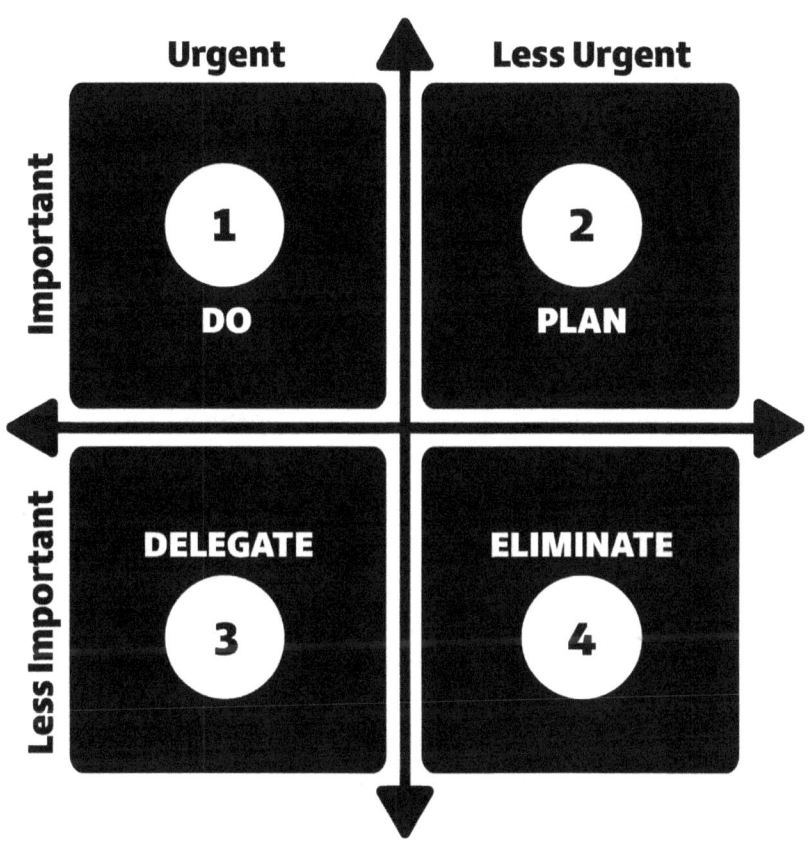

The Immeasurable

As difficult as each of my caregiving situations were and for as many times as I sat in the bathroom and sobbed that I didn't think I could do it even another day, I would not trade this profound, intimate, loving time I had with my mother, my husband, and even my dad for anything. They each had a comfortable, dignified death, and I know my love and hard work contributed to that.

So, because of the nature of the vision—a comfortable, dignified end of life for your care recipient; a smooth transition from caregiver to griever; and an emotionally, mentally, spiritually, and physically healthy future for you, the family caregiver—taking note and making the most of the immeasurable is one of the most significant challenges and rewards for a family caregiver.

I think about the times that Bob and I had moments of intimacy. Times we cried together. Times I held him while he cried. Similarly, there were times I *could* have had angry, frustrated responses—and did not. I cherish those memories—both types. The times I breathed in his scent before he died, and the times after he died when I leaned into his closet, took a deep breath, and continued to take in his scent. The lines in his hands. Sometimes, while rubbing his head to comfort him, I would concentrate on the feeling of his skin under my fingertips to remember it later. I happened to take a photo of his hand a few weeks before he died. It is one of the pictures I keep to myself and look at frequently. I loved his hands, and I feel so fortunate to have the photo.

Remember to notice and cherish the immeasurable. This part of caregiving is for the well-being of the future you. There will be grief when your care recipient becomes more ill and dies. There is a difference between grief rooted in love and grief rooted in despair. Grief rooted in love is beautiful, and if you are lucky enough to love someone, you will experience grief rooted in love when they die. Grief rooted in despair, in my experience and observations, comes from regret.

By keeping the vision top of mind and holding space for the immeasurable, you are working toward grief rooted in love rather than regret or remorse.

4

Facility, Environmental Services & Supplies

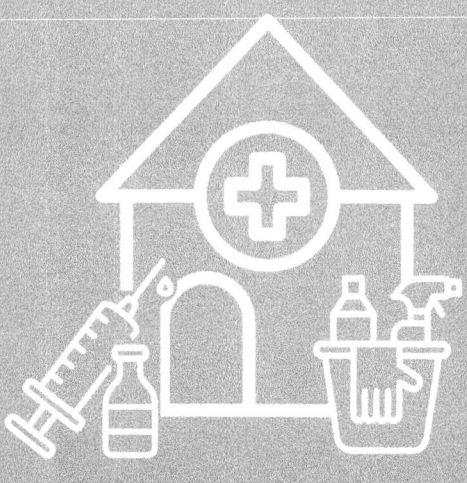

New Message
To: Family Caregiver
Subject: The shower incident

Dear Caregiver,

Bob was just a couple days away from his death, on home hospice, barely able to walk on his own, when I discovered him in the shower. I, fully clothed, quickly got in with him. I held him with one arm and washed him with my other hand as thoroughly as I could. I was so startled and scared I was crying and swearing under my breath the whole time. I am certain it was only a few minutes, but it felt like an hour. When I finished washing him, I used that now free hand to turn the water off, still holding him upright with the other arm. The instant the water was off, my non-verbal, actively dying, beloved husband whispered, "Cold, I'm cold." My heart was breaking and is again as I share this story with you.

The six-by-six-inch curb of our shower may as well have been Mt. Everest, because I could not get him over it. I tried to lift him, but he was too heavy. He could not lift a foot to try and step over the curb, and the flooring in our bathroom was made of an exceptionally slippery material that really should never have been used for a bathroom floor. By this time, I was crying and panicked, thinking we were both going to fall and neither one of us would realize the vision of a peaceful, dignified, death.

I whispered to him, "Bob, you have to help me get you out of here." He turned and positioned himself where I could ease him into a seated position on the bench of his walker, which, thankfully, I had pushed up to the shower door and set the brake upon discovering him in the shower. I dried him off, pushed him into the bedroom and sort of dumped him into the bed, then covered him up—he was already asleep. He was sleeping about twenty-two hours a day at that point in his dying process. I went around to the other side of the bed, got in with him, and sobbed with relief.

We had sold our house, downsized, and moved into a condominium in preparation for Bob's death and my survivorship. We had not had time to fix the bathroom floor and the shower curb to be safer and easier.

I am crying as I write this on the seventh anniversary of Bob's death. This is a painful story for me to recall, much less share. I do it for you in hopes it will help you see that the details of the physical environment or facility are of paramount importance as you see caregiving through the leadership lens.

And I share it because I am with you; I want you to benefit from experiences beyond your own. I know how isolating it feels to be a family caregiver.

I have been where you are, I understand, and I know you can do this.

With love and support,

—jennifer

Just as when you moved into your first apartment and realized certain staples you took for granted in your childhood home—the broom, the doormat, the shower curtain—did not come standard with the rent, we tend to take our homes and the items in them for granted in caregiving. Starting to see family caregiving through a leadership lens, specifically a *health care* leadership lens, we realize that the home as facility, the environment we keep within it (a.k.a. housekeeping), and the supplies we need are crucial parts of the minute-to-minute work as well as the long-term big picture of family caregiving.

The contents of this section:

- Home as Facility
- Medication Management
    - Reference: Medications List
    - Reference: Daily Medications Schedule
- Environmental Services (Housekeeping)
- Supplies
- Transport
- Admissions to Professional Facilities
    - Nights, Weekends & Holidays in Professional Facilities

Home as Facility

A key function within the purview of health care leadership is facilities management. A hospital is a 24/7/365 operation year after year after year. It is not just that it must work all the time. If parts of it don't work, people could die prematurely.

Wherever your care recipient resides, that domicile is just like a hospital or health care residence: It never closes. All basic aspects of the physical plant—including utilities, supplies, and environmental services—must be fully functional at all times.

An effective family caregiver recognizes this and leads the implementation and maintenance of systems and technology that will support full functionality throughout the home 24/7/365.

An occupational therapy consultation or home safety assessment will help ensure the residence is safe for your care recipient. Rebuilding Together, the Administration on Aging, and the American Occupational Therapy Association have created a comprehensive checklist to help make your care recipient's domicile as safe as it can possibly be. Visit aota.org and search for "rebuilding together safe at home checklist" to download the complete document.

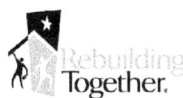

Safe AT HOME
Checklist

Created in partnership with the Administration on Aging and the American Occupational Therapy Association

Rebuilding Together
1899 L Street NW, Suite 1000
Washington, DC 20036
800-473-4229
www.rebuildingtogether.org

Rebuilding Together has long recognized that greater attention must be given our elderly population, so they may age-in-place and safely in their homes. We have also built lasting national partnerships with Area Agencies on Aging, AARP, American Occupational Therapy Association, National Association of Home Builders, National Council on Aging, and others.

Use this list to identify home safety, fall hazards and accessibility issues for the homeowner and family members. Home safety, fall prevention and accessibility modification interventions on the reverse side of this page can help prioritize your work. Underline or use a highlighter to note problems and add comments.

1. **EXTERIOR ENTRANCES AND EXITS**
   - Note condition of walk and drive surface; existence of curb cuts
   - Note handrail condition, right and left sides
   - Note light level for driveway, walk, porch
   - Check door threshold height
   - Note ability to use knob, lock, key, mailbox, peephole, and package shelf
   - Do door and window locks work easily?
   - Are the house numbers visible from the street?
   - Are bushes and shrubs trimmed to allow safe access?
   - Is there a working door bell?

2. **INTERIOR DOORS, STAIRS, HALLS**
   - Note height of door threshold, knob and hinge types; clear width door opening; determine direction that door swings
   - Note presence of floor level changes
   - Note hall width, adequate for walker/wheelchair
   - Determine stair flight run: straight or curved
   - Note stair rails: condition, right and left side
   - Examine stairway light level
   - Note floor surface texture and contrast
   - Note if clutter on stairway

3. **BATHROOM**
   - Are sink basin and tub faucets, shower control and drain plugs manageable?
   - Are hot water pipes covered?
   - Is mirror height appropriate, sit and stand?
   - Note ability reach shelf above, below sink basin
   - Note ability to step in and out of the bath and shower
   - Can resident use bath bench in tub or shower?
   - Note toilet height; ability to reach paper; flush; come from sit to stand posture
   - Is space available for caregiver to assist?

4. **KITCHEN**
   - Note overall light level, task lighting
   - Note sink and counter heights
   - Note wall and floor storage shelf heights
   - Are under sink hot water pipes covered?
   - Is there under counter knee space?
   - Is there a nearby surface to rest hot foods on when removed from oven?
   - Note stove condition and control location (rear or front)
   - Is there adequate counter space to safely prepare meals?

5. **LIVING, DINING, BEDROOM**
   - Chair, sofa, bed heights allow sitting or standing?
   - Do rugs have non-slip pad or rug tape?
   - Chair available with arm rests?
   - Able to turn on light, radio, TV, place a phone call from bed, chair, and sofa?

6. **LAUNDRY**
   - Able to hand-wash and hang clothes to dry?
   - Able to safely access washer/dryer?

7. **BASEMENT**
   - Are the basement stairs stable and well lit?
   - Is there any storage of combustible materials?

8. **TELEPHONE AND DOOR**
   - Phone jack location near bed, sofa, chair?
   - Able to get phone, dial, hear caller?
   - Able to identify visitors, hear doorbell?
   - Able to reach and empty mailbox?
   - Wears neck/wrist device to obtain emergency help?
   - Is there an answering machine?
   - Is there a wireless phone system?

9. **STORAGE SPACE**
   - Able to reach closet rods and hooks, open bureau drawers?
   - Is there a light inside the closet?

10. **WINDOWS**
    - Opening mechanism at 42 inches from floor?
    - Lock accessible, easy to operate?
    - Sill height above floor level?
    - Are storm windows functional?

11. **ELECTRIC OUTLETS AND CONTROLS**
    - Sufficient outlets?
    - Are there ground fault outlets in kitchen and bathroom?
    - Light switch at the entrance to each room
    - Outlet height, wall locations
    - Low vision/sound warnings available?
    - Extension cord hazard?
    - Are there any uncovered outlets or switches?

12. **HEAT, LIGHT, VENTILATION, SMOKE, CARBON MONOXIDE, WATER TEMP CONTROL**
    - Are there smoke/CO alarms and a fire extinguisher?
    - Are Thermostat displays easily accessible and readable?
    - Note rooms where poor light level exists
    - Able to open windows; slide patio doors?
    - Able to open drapes or curtains?
    - Note last service date for heating/cooling system
    - Observe temperature setting of the water heater

Visit aota.org and search for "rebuilding together safe at home checklist" to download the complete document.

Medication Management

There are few more serious aspects of health care leadership than medication management. All medications are an expense to an operation, so if they get lost or diverted, it is money lost. Some medications are controlled substances, including narcotics. If controlled substances get lost or diverted, it is a money loser *and* may result in investigations, license revocation, and perhaps even prison, not to mention potential harm to those who end up using them illegally.

Depending on your care recipient's diagnosis and/or their disease progression, some of the medications in the home may have a street value of more than five times that of cocaine—a serious temptation for diversion.

Remember the vision, the future you. You do not want to jeopardize a future endeavor because of a medication diversion incident on your record. You do not want to regret having failed to manage medications, causing another household member or visitor risky access to narcotics and other controlled substances for recreational use or sale.

And none of the above speaks to the importance of properly administering the medications for their given purpose. There are adverse effects, side effects, dosing requirements, and the potential for human error. Because of these risks, along with the risk of diversion, most hospitals and other professional facilities use an automated medication dispensary system called Pyxis, and most clinics and physician practices have strict protocols about prescribing.

An up-to-date medications management system is essential to your role as family caregiver and leader because it is necessary for smooth cross coverage if/when someone else must take over or fill in for you.

There is a Pyxis-like automated medications dispensary system for the home called Hero Health that can be found at HeroHealth.com. Some health insurance companies and pharmacies have apps and systems for medication management. If you are going to use one of those, confirm that there is a way to share access to the account for cross coverage or delegation.

If you want or need a lower-tech solution to medication management, create and keep an up-to-date medications list and schedule. Include over-the-counter medications and any supplements. You can do this on paper or in a spreadsheet program or app.

Establish a schedule for administering medications, set timers, and be diligent about giving medications on time. Create a reference sheet on what each medication is for and when it is given. Update and replace these documents as things change. The following two pages provide sample layouts for these tools to get you started.

And, when delegating caregiving, remember the value and risks of medications. Lock up everything except what will be needed during a temporary caregiver's coverage time.

- Many medications have more than one name (such as a brand name and a generic name); include them all.
- List vitamins, supplements, and over-the-counter medications, as well as prescriptions.
- Some medications are only given "as needed," which health care professionals refer to as "PRN," which stands for "*pro re nata*," Latin for "as circumstances arise."
- Keep the medication containers provided by the pharmacy. There is important information on the labels.
- If a medication is discontinued by the physician, put a thin line through the entry with the date it was stopped so that you may still reference the information if needed in the future.
- Keep an up-to-date version of this medications list in the portable medical record you keep with the go bag, as discussed in the Strategy & Planning section.

Reference: Medications List

Patient Name: _____ Date of Birth: _____

Medication Names	Prescribing Provider	Date Started	Dose/Freq	AM or PM	Purpose of Medication

Reference: Daily Medications Schedule Daily Medications Schedule for the Week of _____

Patient Name: _____ Date of Birth: _____

Time Taken [AM]	Medication	Dose	Notes

Time Taken [PM]	Medication	Dose	Notes

In the "Notes" column, list any medication effects the temporary caregiver should be aware of, such as "may cause sleepiness," along with other corresponding daily routine activities, such as naps and meals, to help with the continuity of care.

Medications can be a charged and emotional topic. But effective leaders inspire people to peak performance, even in difficult or emotionally charged situations, by sharing reasons and explanations and confirming understanding and acceptance. So, you may want to add a column that lists what the substance treats so that temporary caregivers understand the "why" of administering the medication. You may also want to add an introductory sentence or two such as:

Dear _____,

*Thank you for helping us out this week. I have created this schedule to empower you with the latest routine and medications schedule so that, as caregiver, you and **(care recipient name)** may benefit from continuity in care and have the information you need. Please feel free to make notes so that when I resume caregiving, I will benefit similarly.*

With gratitude,

Environmental Services (Housekeeping)

Helping environmental services (a.k.a. housekeeping) staff members understand the importance of their work is something I put considerable effort into in all the health care leadership positions I hold.

Environmental services are of paramount importance in health care. Dust bunnies in the corner do not instill confidence in patients and their families. Moreover, mess can contribute to illness and injuries. Dust and dander can worsen respiratory conditions, and an orthopedic injury resulting from tripping over something on the floor is at best problematic and at worst extremely serious.

A clean, organized space will also give you, the family caregiver, a greater sense of order and control. Opportunities for order and control are few and far between for the family caregiver; take advantage of this one. Do not think housekeeping is just one of those things that will take care of itself. It is a mark of quality that can be perceived by everyone involved, and it can indeed affect a care recipient's quality of life and comfort in death.

Enlist volunteers to help, or consider a budget allocation for regular cleaning services. Be sure to lock up medications when visiting cleaners and other helpers are present.

Supplies

For the CEO and the family caregiver, never running out of critical supplies is essential. Keeping costs down is equally important. Health care organizations have inventory supply management software that allows them to operate a just-in-time (JIT) supplies provision process. JIT processes keep expenses down by ordering and purchasing only right before a supply runs out and only if needed. Many apps and services are available to the family caregiver to ensure smooth inventory levels.

Resources for home supplies management:

- Pharmacy app
- Smart speakers
- Grocery store app
- Instacart app
- Cleaning supply apps and memberships
- HeroHealth.com
- ByramHealthcare.com

Some of these apps and local businesses have gift registries and wish lists so that you can have other family members and friends share in the expenses and spend on stuff you *need* rather than waste money on kind but frivolous gifts.

Don't forget to seek out local options such as durable medical equipment (DME) stores and pharmacies. These local options may enable a valuable connection with an experienced professional human who gets to know you and the situation with your care recipient.

Transport

One key function of oversight for the health care CEO is transport, or how patients move within a hospital or facility from their room to places like imaging or surgery departments. Have you ever wondered why hospital staff insist on a wheelchair all the way through the front door to the car for a patient who is well enough to be discharged from a facility? Fall prevention is the answer.

Falls can make a difficult situation far worse. At the very best, falls in a health care situation are traumatic. As caregivers, we don't need any more stress and trauma. More often, if an ill, weakened, or older person falls, physical injury will occur. With illness, treatments, and age, bones become brittle and joints arthritic. A fall can have an adverse effect on the vision of a peaceful, comfortable death. For example, the twelve-month mortality rate following a hip fracture in a healthy sixty-five-year-old is 22–29 percent.[9] Because the most common intervention following a hip fracture is surgery, the vision of a peaceful death at home is jeopardized following a hip fracture. Falls are serious stuff.

---

9 S. Haleem, L. Lutchman, R. Mayahi, J. E. Grice, and M. J. Parker, "Mortality Following a Hip Fracture: Trends and Geographical Variations over the Last 40 Years," *Injury Journal* (March 2008).

Admissions to Professional Facilities

An effective leader knows that when an enterprise is faced with profound external change, the internal response must be equal to or greater than those external factors to come through it successfully. In family caregiving, a hospital or facility admission is just such a significant external change. At first, it may seem like you can kick back and share the caregiving load, but the burden is equal or greater because:

- An admission means the care recipient's condition has become more acute or complex.
- There are suddenly more people involved. They work in shifts and often use unfamiliar medical jargon and abbreviations.
- There are a lot of moving parts, protocols, regulations, and laws that facilities must adhere to.
- Professional caregivers (physicians, nurses, etc.) often hyper focus on the patient and discount the role of the family caregiver.

Apply a facilitative, participative, and inspirational approach when a leadership role is not explicit (the professional caregivers do not know you are the CEO). Here are some ideas that may help you to be more facilitative when your care recipient is in the hospital or another facility:

- Introduce yourself to everyone who comes into the room. Learn their name (and position) and use it in conversation whenever possible.
- Be cognizant of agency. Most people who are ill or injured enough to be admitted to a facility have compromised agency, leaving the family caregiver to assert on their behalf. If, however, your care recipient is cognitively clear, they need to be a part of conversations and decisions.
- Take notes or ask to record conversations on your device.
- Listen without interruption.
- If you need additional information to understand something

clinical, use reputable reference tools on the internet, such as WebMD, the facility's own website, or the sites of the Mayo Clinic, Cleveland Clinic, or a respected relevant specialty or diagnosis organization.
- Respectfully assert your role by asking how you can help or what to watch out for.
- Understand that most health care workers feel grossly overburdened and unappreciated. Even though you may feel the same, anything you can do to make them feel less so, such as expressing your compassion for their burden, bringing a box or plate of treats and offering them to each who enters the room, or delivering treats to the nurses' station, will help.
- If a conversation isn't going well, stop and start over.
- Ask for clarification. And keep asking until you understand.
- Use the teach-back method (discussed in the Team & Resources section) to make sure you have properly understood.
- Express gratitude (even when you don't feel it 100 percent).

Remember to take the medical records and go bag (referred to in the Strategy & Planning section) with you to all admissions—and even to outpatient health care services, such as imaging and physician visits, that *might* turn into admissions.

Nights, Weekends & Holidays in Professional Facilities

While a hospital, skilled nursing, or rehabilitation facility is a 24/7/365 operation, that does not mean it always operates the same way.

During what the rest of the world calls the business week—8:00 a.m. to 5:00 p.m. Monday through Friday—there are many more professionals and administrative staff present in the facility. There is a hustle and bustle that simply does not exist during nights, weekends, and holidays.

Nights, weekends, and holidays are different. The leadership of the entire C-suite team and several hierarchical layers of management and administration are not present. Administrative questions and emergencies that cannot wait until the next business day are covered by the designated house supervisor and/or on-call administrator.

Nights are typically quiet and uneventful. If you leave your care recipient's room at the end of visiting hours and return in the morning, that time is usually managed successfully by a reduced staff.

The reduced staff over weekends and holidays, however, may have an impact on the level of attentiveness to a care recipient's needs. When I have had a care recipient in the hospital on weekends or holidays, I've tried to have a friend, a family member, or another stakeholder stay with the care recipient throughout, perhaps overnight depending on the circumstances, even if it means we must take shifts.

Occasionally, it may be necessary to hire a private caregiver to stay in your care recipient's room overnight or during the day when no one else can cover. If you need to hire a professional caregiver to stay in a care recipient's facility room overnight and don't know where to find one, ask in your community (perhaps on social media), or consult the facility's social worker, nursing aide, or patient advocate about reputable services.

5

Self-Management

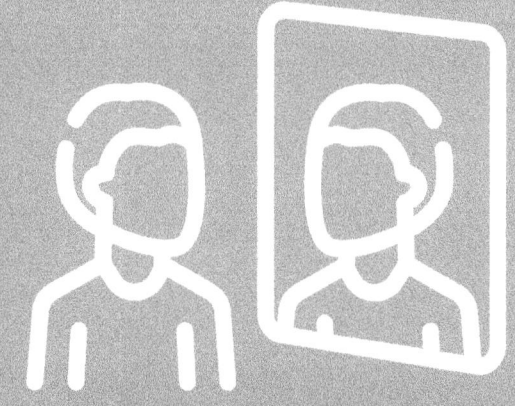

New Message
To: Family Caregiver
Subject: Never-ending quest

Dear Caregiver,

I wish I felt more confident about my own self-management as I begin this section. I don't. I did and do my best, but personal development is a never-ending quest, and caregiving, then grieving, add heavy layers to the challenge.

I have been fortunate enough to access a professional therapist for the last twenty years. When I started going to therapy, it was not as mainstream and accepted by society as it is now. I did not feel that I could share the fact with friends and colleagues, nor, at the time, did I feel I could submit the expense through my employer-provided health insurance; I feared I might be labeled unfit for leadership.

Still, since the beginning, I have felt therapy is the best time and money I have ever spent, both personally and professionally. In the last ten years, I have been able to share that belief openly.

I have gone to two therapists over time. The first one, whom I worked with on and off for several years, helped me see myself and my personal history and patterns in a way that propelled my personal development. When Bob was diagnosed, however, that therapist was no longer a fit. She had helped me so much in the years prior, but despite the fact that Bob and I knew, perhaps better than most, that he was dying, she offered only unrealistic tropes about his prognosis. I was lucky enough to find another therapist who had been a caregiver to her late partner who had died following an illness.

Still, I confess, the top three self-management issues I continue to work on are:

1. Setting and maintaining boundaries.
2. Recognizing and celebrating myself and my achievements.

3. Being as kind, gentle, and forgiving with myself as I am with others.

I share all of this with you because I can now. Also, I don't think I am an outlier here, and I know it always helps me to learn that others are facing some of the same challenges I am or have.

If you can access professional help that fits you and your situation, please do. The ROI on consulting someone who has some objectivity and experience along with unfettered support for *you* and *what is best for you* is invaluable to a family caregiver. The palliative care social worker can be a resource or recommend someone. There are also technologically supported therapy resources, such as BrightSide and Talkspace. Help Texts is a service that sends supportive, informed texts to family caregivers (as well as grievers), with a supportive network in case of emergency. Many faith-based organizations, employer assistance programs, and other community resources offer group support or counseling for caregivers at low or no cost.

In addition, I offer you this self-management section. I hope these offerings help you to know that someone else has experienced similar struggles, and that some tried-and-true methods have helped.

If nothing else, please know that I see you, understand you, support you, and love you.

—jennifer

Self-care involves actions and practices that enhance our physical, mental, emotional, and spiritual well-being and bring us comfort and delight.

Self-management is about actions and practices that navigate, regulate, and manage our behaviors, emotions, and resources effectively toward overall personal and professional goals. Self-management is much broader than self-care.

The mission and vision have you managing yourself in the now, in the near future, and in the long term. This is not self-care, this is self-management; it's bigger and more serious.

The contents of this section:

- Water, Food & Rest
- No Self-Care Shaming
- Past, Present & Future Self
- What-Ifs
- Managing the Negative Thought Spiral
- Intensity Assessment Tool
- Emotional Self-Awareness
    - The Feelings Wheel
    - Feelings & Needs Inventory
- Red Phone Friends
- Personal Outlets
    - Creating
    - Nature
    - Exercise
    - Social Media

Water, Food & Rest

Let's start with the basics. And while this is (*duh*) obvious, it still sneaks up on me. The family caregiver, and to some degree the CEO, must see the momentary through as intently and thoroughly as they see the overall mission and move toward the vision. From the mundane to the intense, seeing the momentary through requires clear thinking and a sound disposition. These cannot be achieved without the basics—water, food, and rest.

We know that the body is 60 percent water and that the brain itself is 75 percent water. A recent study[10] indicates the ill effects of dehydration on metabolism, body temperature, and blood pressure, as well as cognitive performance and mood.

We know from Snickers ads that there is such a thing as "hangry," which is a combination of being hungry and angry that is cured by eating. And of course, we have all had more than one bad day following a fitful night's sleep.

My late husband used to remind himself and me never to get too hungry or too tired. Fatigue, hunger, and even the slightest dehydration can make everything seem like it's falling apart. Sure enough, when I find myself in a state of sitting-still overwhelm, I usually discover that if I drink some water, get something in my stomach, and/or rest for even five minutes, I feel more centered and less likely to completely lose my cool.

I use the term "sitting-still overwhelm" to refer to feeling overwhelmed for no immediate or apparent reason. I am not talking about being overwhelmed in the throes of disaster. It's the times when your mind is spinning into the negative unprovoked, or when you find yourself asking, "What in the world is wrong with me?" In just these times, some water, a snack, and/or even a five-minute rest will bring some focus and clarity.

---

[10] N. Zhang, S. M. Du, J. F. Zhang, and G. S. Ma, "Effects of Dehydration and Rehydration on Cognitive Performance and Mood among Male College Students in Cangzhou, China," *International Journal of Environmental Research and Public Health* (May 2019).

Pro tip: Sleep is important for both leadership and caregiving, yet thoughts and ideas come at all hours. Keep a pad and pen near your bed so that when you wake in the middle of the night with an important thought, you can easily, quietly, and quickly make a note of it in a way that does not awaken you any further, thereby allowing you to go back to sleep. I don't use a device for this, because picking up a device can be distracting, and looking at a screen stimulates my brain in a way that makes it less likely that I will be able to return to sleep quickly.

No Self-Care Shaming

Now that we have established there is a difference between self-care and self-management and that the basics—water, food, and rest—are the core of both momentary and longer-term, effective self-management, let's acknowledge that most of the world thinks in terms of self-*care*. Furthermore, "self-care" has become a pithy phrase that equates to an excuse to eat a piece of chocolate cake or have a pedicure.

My pet peeve is what I call self-care shaming. This is when people with little or no family caregiving experience offer directives in a finger-wagging tone like:

"Make time for yourself."

"Schedule a mani-pedi."

"You won't be able to take care of your person if you don't take care of yourself."

That last one is a big eye roll for me. Many people—especially doctors and nurses—say it. While it is indeed true, family caregivers do not need to be reminded of this. We *know* better than anyone that if we are not well enough to care for our person, no one else will. Some days the best self-care we can do is four consecutive deep breaths.

I don't know how to get the world to stop self-care shaming family caregivers. When I can, I try to teach health care professionals that when a family caregiver is in tears during a clinic or hospital visit, a lecture or even a comment about self-care is contraindicated. We know that if we don't take care of ourselves, we won't be able to take care of our care recipient. In all likelihood, that is not why we are crying. I encourage family caregivers to pay no attention to the self-care shaming and/or to try to articulate the specifics of their own underlying issue or need.

JUST SAY NO TO Self-Care Shaming

Past, Present & Future Self

No matter how you came into the position of family caregiver, you bring your own past, your current being, and your future self with you. This is a fact. With family caregiving, it is especially important to recognize one's past self, because 89 percent of family caregivers care for a spouse or parent,[11] which means, likely, your personal history is entwined with your care recipient's.

Because my only sibling, David, died in an accident when I was eighteen and he was thirteen, my relationships with my parents were profoundly affected. When the hospitalist first told me that my mother had an aggressive, terminal cancer, I knew that deep down learning she was dying was going to provide her some solace. She had lived with the grief of my brother's death for nearly twenty years, and she was tired. I also realized that I would not be her sole caregiver for years to come, because she would die young. That is an example of both of our past selves and my future self contributing to my thoughts and feelings.

When my husband was diagnosed with terminal cancer, I suffered from anticipatory grief, because I had already lost my brother and my mother, and I knew how much it was going to hurt when my husband died. Before I really named and understood my own anticipatory grief, it befuddled me with a general unnamed anxiety and lack of focus. After a friend helped me to identify it, I was able to read about anticipatory grief and accept that a factor from my past was influencing me as I cared for my husband.

In the table that follows, identify elements and prevailing emotions from your past and present that may be affecting your caregiving experience. If your care recipient is willing and able, ask them to do the same. If your care recipient is unable or unwilling, perhaps you can make some notes on their behalf.

Notice that there is a designated space for your future, but not for

---

[11] National Alliance for Caregiving (NAC) and AARP, *Caregiving in the US 2020*.

your care recipient's. This is because the care recipient most often precedes the caregiver in death. There is a space for the care recipient to share their wishes for your future after they have died.

Use this exercise to identify and share important elements of the past and current situation, as well as their potential impact on your future. Perhaps you will make two copies, each complete your part, and have a discussion or ongoing conversation about these factors as part of your relationship. Or you could leave the paper out of it completely and use some or all of the prompts as conversation starters: "Mom, what about our past relationship do you think is impacting this caregiving situation now?" "Do you have any thoughts or wisdom for me about my future after your death?"

Your present self may be affected by specific changes that disease or circumstances have had on your relationship with your care recipient. Perhaps addiction, poor choices, dementia, or some other factor has affected the situation and your present self. This was certainly a factor in my caregiving relationship with my father. I could not have done this exercise or had these conversations with him. Still, this is about *your* self-management, so maybe as the family caregiver you will choose to simply complete the exercise for yourself alone—to manage and influence your present and future self only.

Self-awareness is an essential part of effective caregiving and leadership. The purpose of this prompt is to enhance your self-awareness as it pertains to your caregiving and your future. Use it or skip it to that end.

Past, Present & Future Self

Caregiver			
Past Self Prior to Relationship *(applicable when care recipient is a spouse or friend)*	**Past Shared Relationship**	**Current Shared Relationship**	**Future Self**

Care Recipient			
Past Self Prior to Relationship *(applicable when caregiver is a spouse or friend)*	**Past Shared Relationship**	**Current Shared Relationship**	**Wishes for My Caregiver's Future**

What-Ifs

As a CEO and as a family caregiver I am an overthinker of an Olympic grade. What-ifs (followed by all the possible, terrible things that could happen) are not uncommon for family caregivers. And, honestly, I cannot say that in either position (leader or family caregiver) what-ifs are a complete waste of time, because sometimes they help us anticipate, plan, and prepare. Often, however, the what-if fears become out of control and have an adverse effect on our own well-being.

To neutralize what-if fears, it helps to name them and claim them. So, in the left column on the next page, list your current what-if fears. List them all. Just write them down as they come to mind. When it feels as though you have exhausted all of them, step away from the list. Take some deep breaths. Drink a glass of water or tea.

Next, come back to the list and put a line through those that are especially ridiculous and unlikely. After that, look for those that you feel you need to ask a professional—physician, nurse, lawyer, doula, etc.—about to either eliminate or prepare for. Highlight those. For those that remain without a line through them or a highlight, choose a time when you are well rested, hydrated, and sated to sort out how you might respond if they happen.

Perhaps as or more important, complete the column on the right by listing all of your what-if hopes. Same thing here: Just write them all down as they come to mind. Give yourself some time with this one, because hopes don't seem to pile on naturally the way that fears do. Aim to name as many hopes as you had fears on your original list (*before* you crossed out some of them). Keep going with the hopes.

The aim here is to demonstrate that "What if?" is a neutral question, and that we are capable of naming—perhaps even manifesting—our hopes as easily as our fears. The hopes are not unlike the Universe column of the daily to-do list we covered in the Strategy & Planning section. The Universe list entry I mentioned from near the time of Bob's death said that I wanted him to live through the holidays and die quickly and quietly when the time came. This started as a what-if fear. In mid-December, I started to worry that he was going to die on Christmas. I reframed it as a what-if hope and listed it on the Universe list each day for the last two or three weeks of his life. He died on January 19.

What If . . .	
Fears	Hopes

Managing the Negative Thought Spiral

Sometimes it feels like my brain does its most intricate and productive work when embroiled in the negative and self-criticism. My mind just seems to go into overdrive. One negative or self-deprecating thought leads to another and another and another. I call this the negative thought (downward) spiral, and here is the simple four-step process I apply to overcome it.

1. Recognize that I am experiencing fast and furious negativity and self-criticism.
2. Accept that it is perfectly natural. Estimates are that adults have approximately six thousand thoughts per day.[12] Additionally, there is ample empirical evidence that adults consider negative information far more than positive.[13] That's right: It happens to everyone. I am not an outlier; I am just another adult human.
3. Call yourself by your name and speak to yourself as though you are someone else. For example: "Jennifer, now stop this spiral of negative thinking. Jen, you know this is perfectly natural and entirely unproductive."
4. Slow down and tend to some basic needs like deep breathing, hydration, nutrition, and/or rest. Recognize only the thoughts that are well-founded, reasonable, and/or persistent, and then reframe them.

If these thoughts are about stuff within your control, perhaps put them on the "Me" portion of your to-do list. If you need to assign them to the Universe, reframe them and put them on that list. Perhaps revisit the what-ifs hopes list so you can reframe them and place them there.

If your inner critic is the relentless insomniac that mine is and you

---

12 Julie Tseng and Jordan Poppenk, "Brain Meta-State Transitions Demarcate Thoughts across Task Contexts Exposing the Mental Noise of Trait Neuroticism," *Nature* (July 2020).
13 Amrisha Vaish, Tobias Grossmann, and Amanda Woodward, "Not All Emotions Are Created Equal: The Negativity Bias in Social Emotional Development," *Psychology Bulletin* (May 2008).

need additional help managing your negative thought spirals, consult the short book *Chatter: The Voice in Our Head, Why It Matters, and How to Harness It* by Ethan Kross.

Intensity Assessment Tool

An objective assessment of the situation is an asset to a leader. It's one of the reasons leaders hire outside consultants and advisors.

Archangels (Archangels.me) is an organization that supports and highlights the work that family caregivers do. They have created an assessment tool. It is a series of questions to answer, which will take you ten minutes to complete and will yield an intensity score specific to your caregiving situation. Further, it will let you know whether the degree of intensity has you in the green, which feels manageable; in the yellow, which feels more intense; or in the red, which may well verge on or be overwhelming.

This will give you some objectivity regarding just *how* intense things are overall, rather than how it might feel when you are perseverating or panicking at 3:00 a.m. Remember, an objective measurement of the situation is an asset. Go to Archangels.me to use the intensity assessment calculator and determine the level of your caregiver intensity. Keep the URL handy. You will want to do it again and again as your situation changes.

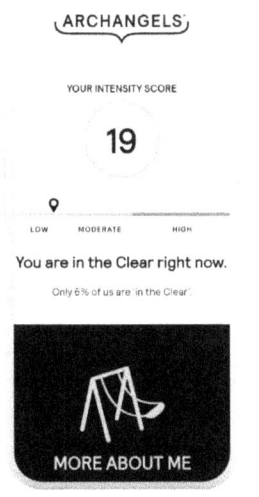 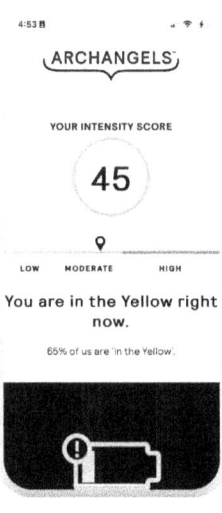 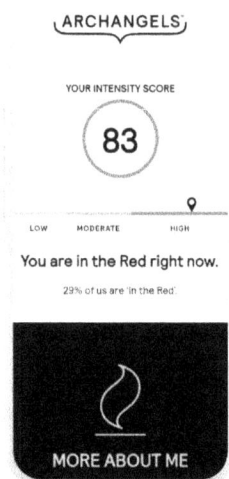

Emotional Self-Awareness

In leadership, emotional self-awareness is important. In family caregiving, it is crucial. Yet the higher the stakes, the more jumbled and unclear our emotions become.

Begin by getting over the idea that there are good or positive and bad or negative emotions. You may like or dislike *experiencing* an emotion, but that does not make the emotion itself bad or good. Each and every emotion stands alone without judgment or qualification as to a value or nature. Suppressing your own anger at having to put a career on hold to take care of someone who wasn't all that nurturing to you in your childhood—because "anger is bad"—will prove a grossly deficient method for dealing with that powerful, pervasive emotion, and will likely harm you in the process.

As caregivers, we need to develop skills at identifying our feelings and sorting out where and when they support and align with the moment, the mission, and/or the vision and where and when we need to more actively manage them so that they are not obstructive. As leaders, we must do all that as we interact with others—and sometimes on behalf of others.

Start by becoming adept at identifying, discussing, and consciously responding to needs and emotions—your own and others'. There are two tools available on the internet to help with this.

The Feelings Wheel

If you search "feelings wheel," you will discover a very useful visual developed by Gloria Willcox, PhD, that organizes a total of seventy-two emotions in a circular chart in six major groups: sad, mad, scared, joyful, powerful, and peaceful. From there it breaks each of those six into another, more specific six feelings, with a third outer circle exploring additional individual emotions.

This approach may help to suss out the details and dimensions of an overall feeling. For example, a general sense you habitually think of as "inferiority" connected to your caregiving situation may be a bit of boredom or even fatigue, which both stem from and feed the core emotion, which is sadness. I know inferiority rears its ugly head with me often when I am feeling lonely and perhaps not as well rested—it is happening to me today as I write this portion of the book! The feelings wheel helps me explore the depths of my own feelings more accurately, which allows me to address them more effectively and communicate with others. It also helps me in doing the same with others in conversations about their feelings.

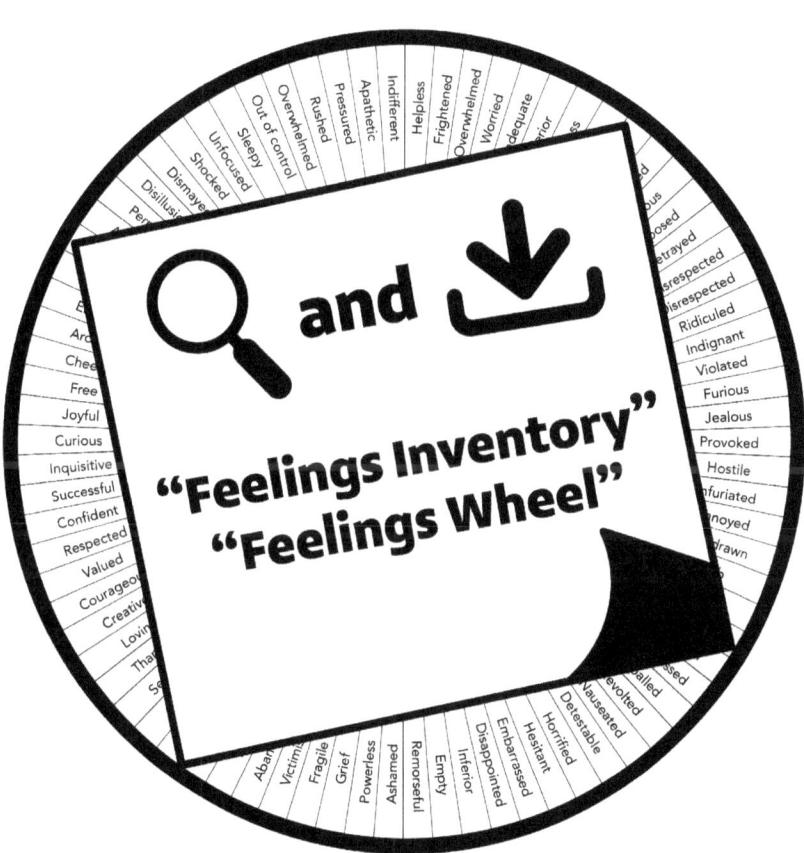

Feelings & Needs Inventory

The second resource can be found as a free download at cnvc.org, the website of The Center for Nonviolent Communication, and is called "Feelings and Needs Inventory." This one comprises three lists.

1. Feelings When Needs Are Satisfied
2. Feelings When Needs Are Not Satisfied
3. Needs Inventory

The first list has eleven headings, each followed by a list of more specific or nuanced terms. The second has fourteen headings, each with a long list of additional or more particular ways of describing the sense or feeling. And finally, the third page is a thorough list of human needs.

Consider the first list of feelings when needs are satisfied and recall the pinpointed positive feedback portion of the Team & Resources section. Pinpointed positive feedback is indeed the most powerful tool in your leadership and communication toolbox. When you find yourself experiencing the feelings associated with your needs being satisfied, note the specifics of how it was achieved. Congratulate yourself for your part, and be sure to provide specified feedback and thanks to anyone else who helped.

The feelings and needs inventory is designed as a starting point for deepening self-discovery as well as our connection with others.

Both the feelings wheel and the feelings and needs inventory are highly accessible ways to develop our emotional awareness. Please download and spend some time with them for self and relationship exploration.

Red Phone Friends

I have many friends, but I only have a couple I feel comfortable calling when I am going nuclear. Those are my red phone friends (RPF).

When you are in a role of great responsibility such as CEO or family caregiver, there just aren't that many people you can call when you are losing your temper, crying uncontrollably, or at a complete and utter loss as to what to do next.

Determine who your red phone friends are. Remember their response must consistently be supportive and calming to you. You need to feel comfortable calling them anytime. You might never call or text in the middle of the night, but you know you could if you needed to.

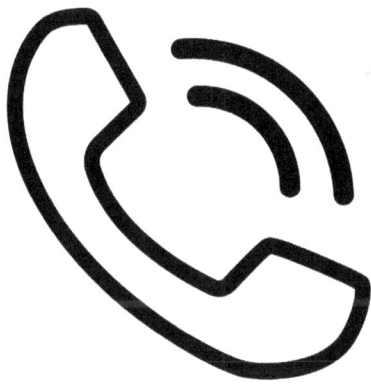

To maintain the relationship and balance, send your RPFs a message of appreciation every now and then, when there is nothing disastrous happening.

Personal Outlets

Outlets, such as exercise, time spent outdoors in nature, creativity, therapy, meditation, journaling, etc., are an essential part of effective self-management for caregivers.

Creating

For me, creating art is my outlet of choice. Some of my digital collages are below and that's how my book *The Hospice Doctor's Widow: An Art Journal of Caregiving and Grief* came about. It was not created to be a book. It was my personal outlet while I was the sole family caregiver for Bob. I continued art journaling for about a year and a half after he died. I did it as part of my self-management. It was about three years after Bob's death that a physician read it and suggested I try to get it published to help other family caregivers and grievers.

Outlets may need to be scaled to fit caregiving responsibilities. That is, there may not be time or space for full-blown studio work. There are several outlets that can indeed be practiced in the limited time and space that caregivers have. If you have an outlet that requires too much time and space during your caregiving, think about ways to scale it down to fit within your caregiving life or replace it with something else that fits.

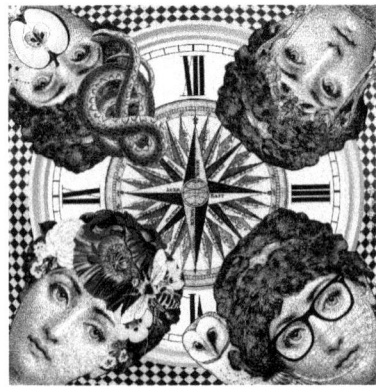
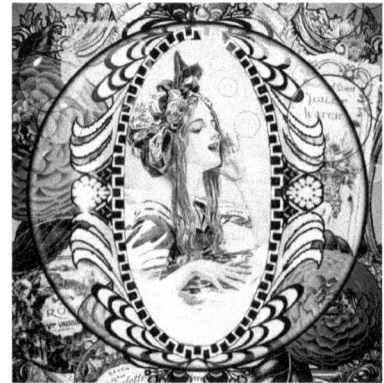

If you think art journaling may be an outlet for you, visit JenniferAOBrien.com/Resources to download my free art journaling prompts and give it a try. If you would like some other ideas for creative outlets that do not require a studio space or significant equipment, some ideas follow.

Creative Outlets

- Knitting
- Puzzles
- Embroidery
- Leisure reading
- Coloring
- Zen doodling
- Drawing
- Watercolors
- Journal writing
- Cross-stitch
- Sewing
- Word games
- Cooking
- Smartphone photography
- Herb gardening
- Miniature making
- Graphic design
- Clay
- Baking
- Card making
- Calligraphy
- Hand lettering
- Collage
- Sketching
- Digital art
- Felting
- Writing/reading poetry
- Crocheting
- Singing
- Beadwork
- Scrapbooking
- Musical composition
- Painting
- Origami
- Papier-mâché
- Notes to friends
- Daydreaming

Nature

Being in nature is a universal outlet. There is a beauty, serendipity, and awesomeness to nature that allows our minds to take a break and our hearts to open. Perhaps your caregiving role does not allow you to do long hikes or camping trips. Scale it down to a daily fifteen-minute walk in the park or backyard. Consider researching some future hiking or camping adventures. Researching, planning, and anticipating can be half the fun sometimes.

Exercise

Some form of physical activity is another universal outlet. It does not have to be hardcore weight training or marathon running. In fact, in the life of a caregiver there is probably neither the time nor the space for either of these efforts. There are, however, shorter runs, apps for yoga and mat exercise, and thirty-, ten-, and even six-minute workouts. Be mindful of not injuring yourself so you don't throw off the caregiving equilibrium. A CEO can work with a broken ankle; a family caregiver probably cannot. Here again, if you are longing to train for and complete big fitness events such as triathlons or tournaments, consider that researching and planning them *for the future* can be an outlet in and of itself.

Social Media

This one is tricky. Sometimes it seems as though zoning out on social media is an outlet. Scrolling can be fun. With the many caregiver support accounts listed at JenniferAOBrien.com/Resources, scrolling can even be useful and educational. Still, scrolling social media is a bit of a roulette game. Sometimes it makes me feel connected, lighthearted, and perhaps even enlightened, while other times I compare myself to others and feel hurt or embittered.

If I only have enough time for a "quickie outlet," rather than look at social media, I play with photo editing and collage apps on my phone, which brings me back to creativity.

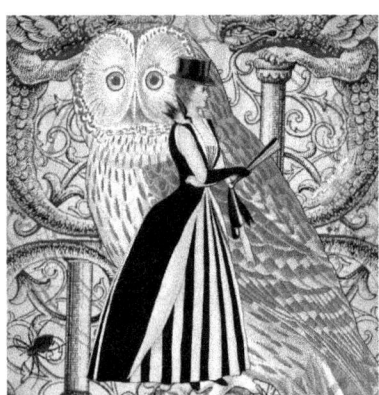
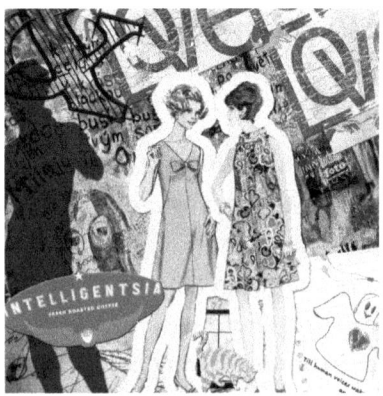

6

Beginning to Realize the Vision

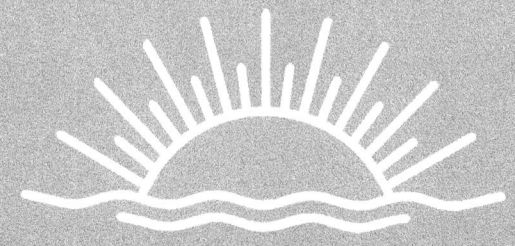

New Message

To: Family Caregiver

Subject: Why didn't the hospice doctor admit himself to hospice sooner?

Dear Caregiver,

Here's where I share with you that my late husband, the hospice and palliative care physician, the man who helped thousands of people see that death was upon them and the comfort and care of hospice services would benefit them, the man who coined the term Precious Time to help people understand death was imminent, did not admit himself to hospice status until just ten days before he died.

As I mentioned in a previous message, it was especially important to Bob that he remain in charge of all the decisions, medications, and specifics. Because it was important to him and I wanted his end of life to be exactly what he wanted, it was important to me. I could see for at least a few weeks that we really needed to put him on a home hospice status. I brought it up a couple of times, and he politely shut down the idea.

Looking back on it, I am certain he had many reasons for waiting. He did not want to die at home, and he was not ill enough to be admitted to an inpatient hospice. He was close with his oncologist, as many cancer patients are, and entering hospice would mean he would no longer be able to see that physician as a patient. And perhaps the biggest reason was that entering hospice care is a very difficult decision, even for an expert in the field. To initiate the transition from evaluating, receiving, and enduring potentially life-prolonging treatments and undergoing imaging and lab work to assess disease progression to simply being comfortable in your own home until you die is not easy, even for the most well-informed and adjusted people.

Bob knew that hospice does not hasten death. Don't let anyone tell you that it does. Bob knew that hospice is not euthanasia or medical aid in dying. Don't let anyone tell you that it is. Bob knew that hospice is not giving up. Don't let anyone tell you that it is. Bob knew that the number one regret of surviving loved ones whose person died in hospice care is that they did not access hospice services sooner.[14] And now you do too.

There is no joy in realizing the family caregiver vision of:

A comfortable, dignified end of life for my care recipient;
a smooth transition from caregiver to griever;
and an emotionally, mentally, spiritually, and physically healthy
future for me, the family caregiver.

But there is certainty in it, at least in the first part: that your care recipient (and you, eventually) will die. Hospice is not the cause of death. Death is not the enemy; suffering is the enemy. Hospice is not giving up; it is when a completely different and final phase of caregiving begins.

I have been through hospice with several loved ones. It *can be* beautiful; it is extraordinarily difficult. If you are thoughtful, deliberate, and present up to and beyond your care recipient's last breath, you will have a greater likelihood of a smooth transition from caregiver to griever and then a healthy future.

I have been where you are. I am where you are headed. I see you. I understand you. I support you, and I love you.

—jennifer

---

[14] "We Wish We Had Known about Hospice Sooner," *Senior Blue Book: Resources for Aging Well* (October 2015).

Remember the three-part vision statement for your use provided at the beginning of the Strategy & Planning section?

> A comfortable, dignified end of life for my care recipient; a smooth transition from caregiver to griever; and an emotionally, mentally, spiritually, and physically healthy future for me, the family caregiver.

Maintaining a leadership perspective during the end of your care recipient's life will not be easy. Realizing a vision of this magnitude takes great work, thought, and intention.

Will your relationship with your care recipient and all the circumstances surrounding their death allow for this vision to be realized? It's not always certain. Their death, however, is entirely certain. While some life-limiting conditions end with an abrupt death, most increase in intensity over time, with the care recipient becoming more ill and incapacitated until their body begins shutting down, and then they die.

As I confessed in my message to you, perhaps one of the most difficult points in the continuum is the decision to enter the hospice phase. Our health care system and our society don't make this decision any easier, because in general we don't openly discuss, prepare for, and accept death. I know of oncologists who see death as defeat or the enemy and therefore will not discuss hospice with patients and families unless forced to. Death will happen with or without the benefits, services, expertise, and experience of licensed hospice professionals.

Hospice means letting the natural course of death take place with some medications, equipment, care, and extra help to make it peaceful and comfortable. Hospice does not hasten death. Hospice is a status, not a place. Most hospice happens in the care recipient's residence. Sometimes hospice status occurs in a health care facility.

Bob used to say, "I have seen hospice deaths thousands of times; the patient is going to be fine. It is the family I worry about." A comfortable, natural hospice death is peaceful for the patient. As someone who has gone through the hospice deaths of numerous family members, I can tell you Bob was right. The dying loved one is ultimately at peace, but it doesn't always feel so peaceful for surviving loved ones.

The average duration of family caregiving is 4.9 years.[15] Perhaps you have been family caregiving for years. You may have started, like I did with Bob, when there was hope your loved one would be cured. While that did not last long for us, the phase where, on the good days, he could work and eat full meals lasted nearly two years. As the family caregiver you are likely to have made keeping your care recipient alive and as well as can be expected your raison d'être for several years. The change from health maintenance family caregiver to hospice/end-of-life family caregiver is, to use CEO language, "a paradigm shift" of extraordinary proportions.

So let's look at some specific facts and observations that will help you make that transition. While you may feel like the change to hospice is a long way off, please read this section now. The transition can arise rather suddenly. You will be better prepared when it does happen if you have read this in advance.

The contents of this section:

- Choice, Change & Discharge
- Admission to Hospice & Insurance Coverage
- Duration
- Access & Listen to the Professionals
- DIY
- Medications
- Precious Time
- The Triad of Certainty

---

15 AARP and National Alliance for Caregiving (NAC), *2020 Family Caregiving Survey.*

Choice, Change & Discharge

You have the right to choose your own hospice provider. You do not have to simply go with your doctor's or hospital's recommendation. While the basic services of hospice are standardized, the quality of care, interaction, organizational culture, family satisfaction survey results, religious affiliation (if any), and for-profit or not-for-profit status make for big differences among hospices. Leaders do their due diligence and shop for the organization that best suits the realization of the mission and the vision. It is never too early to research the hospices that serve your location and determine which might be the best for your care recipient and you.

If you have experienced deficits in hospice care, service, or respect, you have the right to select and change to a different hospice provider. You can come off hospice status at any time. If, for any reason, hospice status and services no longer seem appropriate or beneficial, they can be discontinued.

If you are considering changing hospices or discharge from hospice, please talk with the hospice social worker to learn more about the applicable process so as not to make a big decision hastily or without complete information.

Admission to Hospice & Insurance Coverage

Like a palliative care team, a hospice team is interdisciplinary. It usually includes a physician, nurse, social worker, chaplain, nursing aide, and volunteer.

An admission to hospice will include visits and calls from the nurse, social worker, and chaplain. If the care recipient is covered by Medicare, the team must complete an assessment that includes the patient's medical, emotional, and spiritual needs within five days of the admission. This means a visit from the nurse, the social worker, and the chaplain will happen quickly following the admission. Be prepared for a barrage of calls and visits from these professionals in those first few days.

Medicare, Medicaid, and all other major medical insurances cover all the home hospice services, supplies, and equipment by paying an inclusive per diem rate directly to the hospice. There is typically no co-payment or coinsurance and no other insurance-based out-of-pocket expenses to the patient or family.

Duration

The standard prognosis for hospice is six months or less to live. Some people live longer than six months on hospice, but it is not that common. The overall average length of stay in home hospice is ninety days.[16] For cancer patients the average length of stay in hospice is just nineteen days.[17] So please do not think that you have a full six months with your care recipient once they are admitted to hospice status; the data shows it will be much less, and with cancer it may only be a few days.

You may find yourself wondering, with some frequency, "How long will this go on?" Leaders envision and plan, yet this is one question where all the leadership acumen and experience in the world will not render specifics. When you ask the hospice nurse, "How much longer?" The nurse will answer with phrases such as, "weeks to months," "days to weeks," or "hours to days." Even when your care recipient is actively dying, the process may go on for days, or it may last just a few minutes.

---

16 National Hospice and Palliative Care Organization, *NHPCO Facts and Figures 2022 Edition* (December 2022).
17 Mihir N. Patel, Jonathan M. Nicolla, Fred A. P. Friedman, Michala R. Ritz, and Arif K. Kamal, "Hospice Use Among Patients with Cancer: Trends, Barriers and Future Directions," *Journal of Clinical Oncology* (November 2020).

Access & Listen to the Professionals

Remember, an effective leader hires experienced professionals and then listens to them. Hospice has done this thousands of times. They have honed their skills at anticipating needs. They can see, in a way we cannot, that soon the care recipient will need a hospital bed in the home, a bedside commode, a comfort kit, etc.

Say yes to whatever hospice offers *when* they offer it. Do *not* say, "Oh we're not ready for that yet." Say, "Yes, thank you," and accept it. You may not think you need it. You may think it will upset your care recipient (and it might). Accept it anyway. In a hospice care situation, once you *experience* the need for something, like a piece of equipment or medication, you are past needing it. You are desperate for it, and it can take hours or longer to get it delivered to the home. So just say yes when it is offered so that you will have it on hand if/when the need comes.

If the hospice does not provide them, order Barbara Karnes's end-of-life guideline series for $15 from her website, BKBooks.com. Barbara has been a nurse and world-renowned educator for decades. This little booklet series will be one of your best resources when your care recipient is on hospice status and nearing death. This series takes the many unknowns and provides answers and familiarity, so you can spend more time being with your person and less time wondering what to expect.

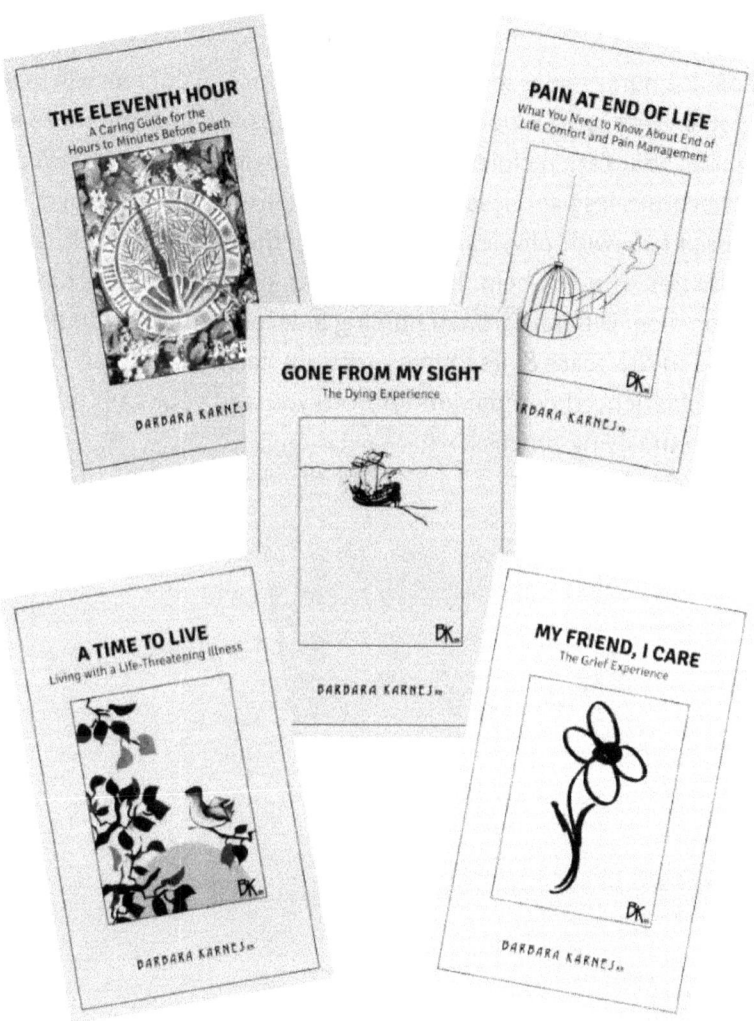

DIY

Hospice has a large DIY (do it yourself) component. It is not 24/7 professional care in your home. However, there is a twenty-four-hour telephone number that you can call with questions or if you have an emergency.

A hospice nurse, aide, social worker, chaplain, or volunteer will make periodic visits to your home. The nurse visits will become more frequent as your care recipient gets closer to dying. As your care recipient becomes less and less able to ambulate and get out of bed, you *will need help* with physical care. Put together a schedule of family and friends who can help. If that is not an option, consider hiring a nursing aide. Different from a nursing aide, an end-of-life doula (described in the Team & Resources section) can be extremely helpful as an experienced companion for both you and your care recipient through the dying process.

Medications

Please refer to the Medication Management portion of the Facility, Environmental Services & Supplies section. With hospice status come both valuable narcotics *and* visitors right there in your home. In other words, a high-risk situation. There is a reason they are called controlled substances; keep them locked up and safe from diversion.

Having said that, as strong as hospice medications may be, know that when you administer them you will not hasten or cause your care recipient's death. Your person is dying. They will die with or without the medication. Caregivers and medications are simply not powerful enough to cause or hasten a death. These medications make the patient more comfortable and restful as they die. And remember, there is always a last dose of medication. Do not second-guess yourself after your care recipient dies by thinking that the last dose of morphine or other medication caused the death. Death happens—with medication for comfort and quiet, or without it.

Your care recipient will likely sleep more and more as they get closer to death. This is perfectly normal, with or without medication. Often the medications make them sleep more soundly and ease agitation.

Precious Time

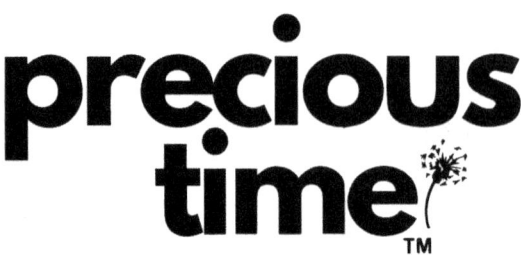

When your care recipient has been admitted to hospice status, you are definitely into Precious Time. Refer to the page about Precious Time in the Strategy & Planning section of this book. Precious Time is when death is likely or imminent. Precious Time is when you lean in and make your love and care known because this person will soon die, then you will go on living. There is no dress rehearsal for the death of your care recipient; you will not get a do-over.

It may be exhausting, scary, or profoundly sad. You may even experience a sense of relief that it will soon all be over. Nevertheless, it is your Precious Time, and you will go on after your care recipient dies and have to live with how you handled that Precious Time.

Those quiet Hollywood deathbed scenes are grossly unrealistic. Take all the soap opera, TV, and film deathbed scenes you remember and disregard them. As hospice educator Barbara Karnes, RN, says, "People don't die like they do in the movies." I will add, "There's no take two."

Because Bob and I talked about his specific end-of-life wishes, I knew that he wanted me and only me there with him as he took his last breath. I was determined to carry out that commitment, even after what I went through with my mom determining that she did not in fact want me present because of how difficult it is to be at the bedside of a loved one. Sure enough, Bob went into that deep, deep sleep and the secretions in his throat produced the very loud breathing known as the death rattle. It was loud; I was so uncomfortable. It was late in the evening, and I knew he was very close to death. I sort of paced around the room not knowing what to do with myself. Finally, I put my pajamas on, pushed the chair right up to the edge of his bed, and settled in. I put my earbuds in and listened to some music that he had introduced me to years prior. I put my hand in his and concentrated on giving him my love, repeating my mantra of "the miracle is peace," and listening to the music. I managed to fall asleep for about an hour, and when I woke, he had died. My hand was still in his and his hand was still warm. Again, just like with my mom, it was surpassingly beautiful and perfect.

So, while death is natural (and thus nothing like what we see in the movies), it is also not always *easy* for loved ones to witness. It certainly hasn't been for me. All I can say is, do everything in your power to get over your fear, sadness, and discomfort.

Express your love. Be fully there.

Your future self, the self who will be grieving the loss, the self who will be looking back, the self who will live with this loss for the rest of your life, will benefit from not carrying the burden of remorse because you were not fully *engaged* in the last days and minutes of your person's life. I chose the word "engaged" because you may not be immediately *with* your care recipient at the bedside when they die. Some people want to spare their loved ones witnessing their death and wait until their family caregiver leaves the room to take their last breath. Some people will wait until they are surrounded by loved ones to take their last breath. In all the times I have been through it with loved ones, I have learned to accept and trust that exactly when they take their last breath and who is with them or not with them is part of something larger than me.

The Triad of Certainty

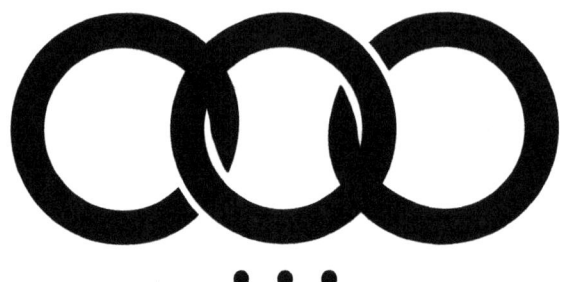

The Triad of Certainty

*At the end of life comes death.
There are no do-overs in end of life.
Changed forever, loved ones remain and remember.*

New Message
To: Family Caregiver
Subject: Encouragement

Dear Caregiver,

We started (in the Introduction) by making lists of words that describe both caregiving and leadership. As we end and think of the adjectives that may accurately describe caregiving for and the death of a loved one, they might be "intense," "rich," "difficult," "profound," "epiphanic," "beautiful" . . . but "easy" will never be one of them.

Nothing about the twenty-two months that Bob was sick and we prepared for his death and my survivorship was easy. But we did it anyway. It was an incredible period and an act of love and intimacy that continues to remind me of our devotion even years later.

The other day (about seven years after his death), I was doing some reorganizing and purging in the condominium that Bob and I downsized to in preparation for his death and my life alone. I had gone through several drawers when I realized there was a flashlight in the top drawer of nearly every table, nightstand, credenza, and chest of drawers in every room throughout the condo.

I had not put those flashlights there. Bob had. He had left a flashlight within reach for me no matter where I was in the apartment. I guess he wanted to be sure that if the power went out, I could just reach for a flashlight and find one at my fingertips.

Like I said, none of it was easy, but all the work we did certainly made it easier on me after he died.

We did it. I did it. And you can do it. You will do it. I know it.

I have been where you are, I understand, I am where you are headed, and it's fine here.

With love and gratitude,

—jennifer

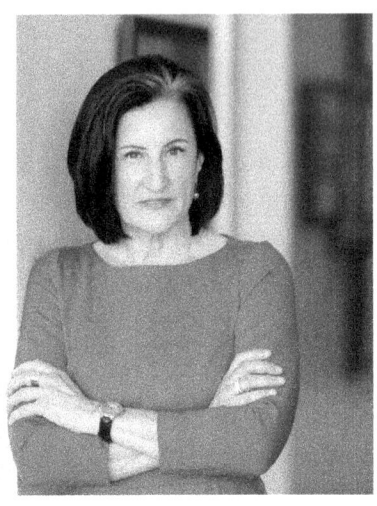

JENNIFER A. O'BRIEN, MSOD, has worked in health care for over thirty-five years, serving as CEO and in administrative leadership positions for medical practices, hospitals, and academic medical centers. She also has personal experience as a family caretaker during her mother's pancreatic cancer, her husband's kidney cancer, and her father's heart and lung disease. A graduate of Boston University and Loyola University–Chicago, she has published over fifty articles in peer-reviewed journals and professional publications and is the award-winning author of *The Hospice Doctor's Widow: An Art Journal of Caregiving and Grief*. Jennifer lives in Little Rock, Arkansas, with her dog, Fido. Learn more at JenniferAOBrien.com.

www.ingramcontent.com/pod-product-compliance
Lightning Source LLC
Chambersburg PA
CBHW070043040426
42333CB00041B/2186